Comprehensive Sports
Injury Management

COMPREHENSIVE SPORTS INJURY MANAGEMENT

From Examination of Injury
to Return to Sport

SECOND EDITION

Jim Taylor, PhD
Kevin R. Stone, MD
Michael J. Mullin, ATC
Todd Ellenbecker, MS, PT
Ann Walgenbach, RN, FNP, MSN

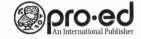
pro·ed
An International Publisher
8700 Shoal Creek Boulevard
Austin, Texas 78757-6897
800/897-3202   Fax 800/397-7633
www.proedinc.com

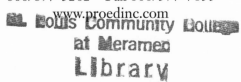

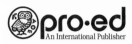

© 2003 by Jim Taylor, Kevin R. Stone,
Michael J. Mullin, Todd Ellenbecker,
and Ann Walgenbach

Library of Congress Cataloging-in-Publication Data

Comprehensive sports injury management : from examination of injury to return to sport
/ Jim Taylor . . . [et al.].—2nd ed.
    p. ; cm.
    Includes bibliographical references and index.
    ISBN 0-89079-891-5
      1. Sports injuries. 2. Sports injuries—Patients—Rehabilitation. I. Taylor,
Jim, 1958–
    [DNLM: 1. Athletic Injuries—diagnosis. 2. Athletic Injuries—
rehabilitation. 3. Athletic
Injuries—surgery. QT 261 C737 2003]
  RD97.C65 2003
  617.1'027—dc21

                                                                   2002031910

This book is designed in Janson Text and OPTIBevis.

Printed in the United States of America

1 2 3 4 5 6 7 8 9 10 07 06 05 04 03

*I would like to extend my appreciation to my coauthors.
Thank you for staying committed, working nights
and weekends, and getting the job done—finally.
And love to my family for always being there.*
—J. T.

*Thanks to the team at the Stone Clinic for their
constant invaluable input to patient care.*
—K. R. S.

*I would like to acknowledge my wife, Kay, and
son, Mitchel, for their patience and support in making
this book possible. I would also like to thank Kevin Stone,
Ann Walgenbach, and the entire staff of the Stone Clinic
for providing the professional and personal environment
from which a substantial part of this book derived.*
—M. J. M.

To Gail, for her patience, love, and understanding.
—T. E.

*I would like to thank my supportive father and
loving husband for generating and perpetuating
my interest in sports, and Dr. Kevin Stone for the opportunity
to take care of a diverse range of patients and athletes.
Finally, thanks to all of the patients who have taught me
so much about being a health professional.*
—A. W.

*Thanks to Susan Steineke, physician assistant, and
Sharon Lang, office manager, both of the Stone Clinic, and
Katherine G. Mullin, R.D., for their contributions to this book.*

Contents

SECTION I
Examination of Injury

CHAPTER 1
Initial Examination 3

CHAPTER 2
Diagnosis and Treatment 25

SECTION IV
Return to Sport

CHAPTER 10
Postrehabilitation Recovery   177

CHAPTER 11
Psychological Concerns of Return to Sport   205

Preface

In recent years, there has been growing awareness and interest among the sports medicine community in considering the whole person in the context of the injury management process. Specifically, sports medicine professionals are increasingly focusing on the impact of a serious injury and the subsequent treatment and rehabilitation on patients physically, psychologically, socially, and logistically. Questions that are often asked include the following:

- What is the typical reaction of injured athletes after learning their diagnosis, and how can I best respond?

- What do patients need to know about surgery to reduce fear and concern?

- What practical things do patients need to know and do to effectively manage themselves during rehabilitation?

- What issues will affect recovery, and how can they facilitate rather than interfere with patients' return to sport?

Sports medicine professionals want to know how they can answer these questions and, more important, how they can use this information with their patients to facilitate the injury management process.

When people sustain an injury, they are forced to participate in a sometimes long and painful process of treatment and recovery. Surgical technology and rehabilitative procedures are so advanced that many individuals can expect to have a full recovery, even from the most serious injuries. Despite these advances, relatively little attention is given to the individual and how the injury affects him or her personally and socially, and how it affects the person's lifestyle. The injured are typically offered little information on how the injury and the injury management process will affect them physically, psychologically, and logistically. The sports medicine professional usually provides limited practical information to assist the injured athlete in preparing for and managing the treatment and rehabilitation process.

Typically, patients are left on their own to learn what kinds of experiences they will have to confront during the course of recovery. This usually results in these issues having a negative rather than positive influence on the quality of the treatment experience. Sports medicine professionals, from the orthopedist to the nurse to the physical therapist or athletic trainer, have a wealth of information that could benefit the injured. However, this information is usually not conveyed to the patient in an organized and practical manner, if at all.

Additionally, the injury management process can often become compartmentalized, not unlike a manufacturing assembly line, in which each person has a specific responsibility, accomplishes the task, and then passes the product on to the next person. From this perspective, workers at different points in the assembly line do not generally have a complete grasp of what has occurred previously or will occur subsequently in the assembly process. This lack of integration can occur for several reasons. Sports medicine professionals are highly specialized and may not receive extensive education about injury management areas outside their own area of expertise. Also, from a practical standpoint, specialists must focus on their primary responsibilities and often do not have the time to devote to other stages in injury management.

We believe, however, that a working knowledge of all aspects of the sports injury management process is essential for sports medicine professionals. Early in the injury process, this knowledge allows them to be a source of information and predictability to their patients. Late in the process, it enables them to understand where the patient has been and to better prepare the patient for what lies ahead.

There are three primary goals of this book: (a) to identify important physical, psychological, and logistical issues that will benefit patients; (b) to provide practical information, guidelines, approaches, and strategies to ensure that the handling of these issues facilitates rather than interferes with the injury management process; and (c) to offer sports medicine professionals a framework with which to provide patients with information about these issues.

Three influential areas are addressed in terms of their effects on day-to-day and long-term injury management: (a) physical issues that the patient will encounter, including injury-specific information such as the nature of the damage, pain, and rehabilitation, in addition to more general physical concerns such as rest and effects on overall health; (b) psychological issues that the patient will face, including anger over the injury, postoperative depression or stress, confidence in the rehabilitation program, motivation to maintain rehabilitation, and loss of identity; and (c) logistical issues related to how the injury will affect the injured person's daily life, for example, how it will affect the person's ability to work, mobility, and satisfaction of basic needs such as bathing and finding transportation.

These concerns are addressed within a chronological framework consisting of a four-stage process of injury management: (a) examination of injury; (b) surgery (when necessary); (c) rehabilitation; and (d) return to sport. Within each stage, issues that most influence the quality of the patient's experience are examined. In addition, practical ways of dealing with each issue are considered, with special emphasis on providing clear information and simple, practical strategies and techniques to manage them most efficaciously.

Interest in this book arose from the authors' divergent yet overlapping professional experiences in injury management. The book is intended for all sports medicine professionals who work in the sports injury management process, including orthopedists, nurses, physical therapists, athletic trainers, psychologists, chiropractors, massage therapists, and other allied health professionals. The objective of this book is to provide the sports medicine professional with comprehensive information for use in the day-to-day work of the injury management process. With this knowledge, sports medicine professionals at every stage of injury management can accomplish two essential goals. First, they can fully understand all of the issues that will affect their patients' recovery experiences. Second, they can ensure that all of these issues are dealt with so as to contribute to, rather than impede, the injury management process.

Introduction

At a fundamental level, the primary focus of sports medicine professionals working with injured athletes is to heal the physical injury. The efforts of these professionals are directed toward the diagnosis, treatment, and rehabilitation of the injury. Recovery from injury is deemed successful if all of the physical parameters associated with the injury have returned to or surpassed their preinjury levels.

The injury management process involves a variety of stages, which may include preliminary diagnosis, initial treatment, testing and evaluation, diagnosis confirmation, development of a treatment plan, surgery, physical therapy, and return to sport. Within these stages, as many as a dozen sports medicine professionals may participate: physicians, orthopedic surgeons, radiologists, imaging technicians, nurses, physician assistants, billing managers, physical therapists, athletic trainers, biomechanists, massage therapists, personal trainers, coaches, nutritionists, and psychologists.

Most often, the involvement of the sports medicine professionals is compartmentalized throughout the injury management process. As injured athletes leave one stage of injury management, they lose touch with the professionals they had worked with previously and are passed on to those who will help them in the subsequent stages of recovery. In addition, there is limited communication between professionals at different stages of the injury management process.

Yet, when athletes sustain an injury, it affects more than just the physical area of trauma. The injury harms the athletes' physical, athletic, psychological, emotional, social, work or school, and daily lives. Although the physical injury can be fully rehabilitated, unless consideration is given to these other areas, there is no guarantee that the athletes will return to full overall functioning and to their highest level of sports performance.

For athletes to recover fully from an injury, every part of their life that is damaged must be rehabilitated. It is essential that sports medicine professionals view the physical injury within the context of a complex set of reactions that athletes experience during the injury management process and which can disrupt many areas of their life. Moreover, these disruptions do not always occur at a specific time or in a predictable way in the injury management process. Rather, disruptions can arise unexpectedly and reappear later in the course of recovery.

To address these issues in a timely and effective manner, sports medicine professionals must see "the big picture" of the entire process, from injury to treatment to rehabilitation to return to sport. They must understand all aspects of injury management and how each can influence the multifaceted reactions of injured athletes during rehabilitation.

Sports medicine professionals must also communicate effectively among themselves across the stages of injury management. This communication allows them to share information, gain perspective and understanding of injured athletes, and develop effective strategies to identify and respond to the multitude of issues that can arise during the course of injury management. It enables sports medicine professionals to see injured athletes as more than just physical injuries and as more than just a point of contact with one specific responsibility in the injury management process.

INTERDISCIPLINARY SPORTS MEDICINE TEAM

An interdisciplinary sports medicine team provides for the diverse needs of injured athletes throughout the injury management process. Members of the team have clearly defined roles that are usually appropriate for a particular stage of injury management. For example, the nurse or physician assistant is primarily responsible for the injured athlete during diagnosis, development of a treatment plan, and surgery, if it is warranted. Similarly, the physical therapist or athletic trainer is primarily responsible during rehabilitation of the injury. The sports medicine physician or orthopedic surgeon often contributes throughout the course of injury management. Additionally, other members of the sports medicine team, such as the massage therapist and the psychologist, may play vital roles in every stage of injury management.

Communication and collaboration between members of the sports medicine team can enhance the continuity and quality of care. For example, concerns that might have arisen early in the injury management process can be followed by a sports medicine team member, and essential information can be passed on to other team members involved later in injury management. This team approach acts to ensure that "all the bases are covered" for injured athletes and that all of their needs are met as they progress through their recovery.

Building an interdisciplinary sports medicine team first involves identifying the diverse concerns and needs of injured athletes over the course of injury management. Primary issues that affect injured athletes include diagnosis, payment for services, logistics, treatment plan, surgery (if warranted), rehabilitation, psychological and emotional difficulties, and return to sport.

A sports medicine team usually involves two levels of involvement. The core team is composed of professionals who play required roles in the injury management process, including the sports medicine physician or orthopedic surgeon, billing manager, nurse, nurse practitioner or physician's assistant, and physical therapist or athletic trainer. These professionals have a necessary part in assisting injured athletes through the stages of injury management.

The support team is composed of professionals whose expertise is not usually integral to the injury management process but who can provide valuable information and skills when specific concerns arise. These include psychologists, biomechanists, massage therapists, nutritionists, personal trainers, and coaches. These professionals can provide specialized support to the core team to address problems that may occur during the course of injury management.

The core team is common to all sports medicine facilities, and member roles are clearly defined. However, involvement of support team professionals is less common. Recruitment of these professionals into the sports medicine team can enable the team to respond promptly and confidently to issues that arise during the injury management process. The core team can identify and recruit support team professionals and create a referral procedure for using them by following the example for finding a qualified psychologist given in Chapter 3.

In addition to the specific roles that the sports medicine team members play in the recovery of injured athletes, they also play a collaborative role that facilitates and augments the primary roles they serve. For example, if a patient facing reconstructive shoulder surgery is experiencing anxiety prior to the procedure, the surgeon or nurse might make a referral to the team's psychologist to assist the patient in overcoming the anxiety and better preparing for the surgery. Similarly, if the physical therapy insurance coverage of an athlete recovering from anterior cruciate ligament (ACL) reconstruction has been exhausted, then the services of a personal trainer might be used to continue the course of supervised conditioning.

It is important for core team members to respect one another's respective fields and to maintain open lines of communication. For instance, if an athlete was referred to physical therapy by an orthopedic surgeon with a prescription for "ACL reconstruction," but the surgeon did not mention a meniscus repair, it is doubtful that the athlete would know that such a procedure had been performed. The treatment approach for an ACL with a meniscus repair is markedly different from treatment not involving meniscus repair. In the absence of this valuable information, the athlete's ultimate outcome might be compromised. The same problem holds true for physical therapists and athletic trainers providing care for patients but not being aware of the physician's preferences. Using the athlete with an ACL reconstruction with meniscus repair as an example, some surgeons would limit the amount of weight bearing, others the range of motion. It is important that the rehabilitation professional be aware of the preferred treatment approach so as to better develop a treatment plan and educate the athlete.

It is also important for support team members to maintain open lines of communication. If, for example, over the course of care for an athlete with a lower back condition, the physical therapist or athletic trainer recognizes that there is more extensive soft tissue restriction throughout the entire midsection, then he or she might refer that athlete to a massage therapist for more extensive manual treatment. The referral should be followed by communication with the massage therapist to discuss findings and the areas on which the massage session should focus. Conversely, the physical therapist or athletic trainer should pay heed to any findings by the massage therapist because they may be relevant to the therapist's or trainer's own treatment of the patient.

The development of optimal treatment algorithms requires a multidisciplinary team approach based on sound principles, research, and communication among core and support team members. Although each practitioner provides an independent service, the more that these services are coordinated, the better the potential outcome. This team approach to injury management maximizes the individual and collective capabilities of the sports medicine team members and allows them to provide injured athletes with the highest quality care possible.

INFORMATION IS POWER

The disruption in the lives of athletes who sustain a serious injury that significantly limits functioning and requires a lengthy rehabilitation is profound and wide-ranging. This disruption hurts athletes psychologically and emotionally and can create uncertainty, doubt, stress, and fear. At the foundation of these negative reactions is simply "not knowing." If sports medicine professionals can relieve the "not knowing," then they will have taken a significant step in responding to those concerns and reducing the negative impact that the injury will have on the athlete.

There is a saying: Information is power. Information and understanding can provide injured athletes with three essential tools for facilitating their recovery from injury: familiarity, predictability, and control. Injured athletes who are familiar with what lies ahead can predict the ups and downs of the injury management process and exert some control over the experience. They will be better equipped to respond positively to the entire process, from the initial exam to their return to sport.

Injuries generate many questions for athletes, which in turn lead to many of the negative reactions that injured athletes may have during the course of their recovery. A fundamental goal for sports medicine professionals in the injury management process is to provide answers. Yet, because most professionals focus on the treatment and rehabilitation of the injury, they do not always provide the answers that injured athletes need to know. Additionally, there may be the presumption that if injured athletes have questions, they will ask. Injured athletes are not always informed consumers, however. Unless they have been injured before, they simply do not know what questions they should ask to make their treatment, rehabilitation, and return to sport as manageable as possible. This is why we believe it is essential that sports medicine professionals take a proactive approach to injured athletes' information gathering.

The injury management process can be greatly facilitated at all levels by having sports medicine professionals answer the questions that their patients should ask if they were informed enough to ask them. To that end, each chapter of this book highlights key questions and answers that sports medicine professionals can provide for their patients.

This proactive approach has many benefits for the sports medicine professional as well as for the injured athlete. For the sports medicine professional, more knowledgeable patients will be more active and willing participants in the injury management process, will be able to provide professionals with relevant information about their injury and rehabilitation, and will place fewer demands on the professionals. Injured athletes will be better equipped to handle the diverse demands of rehabilitation, will respond better to treatment, will be more motivated to adhere to their rehabilitation regimen, will have more timely and complete recoveries, and will be able to return to and perhaps even surpass their pre-injury level of performance.

SECTION I

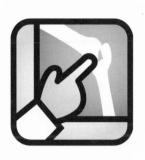

Examination of Injury

CHAPTER 1

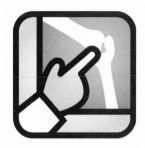

Initial Examination

When newly injured athletes enter the physician's office, they experience a wide range of strong and discomforting thoughts and emotions. The predominant aspect of this first step in the sports injury management process is uncertainty. Injured athletes have many questions and few, if any, answers. These questions can be categorized as either immediate or long-term concerns. Long-term questions include the following:

- How do I find out what is really wrong with me?
- Is there anything we can do to treat my injury now?

During the initial examination, the injured athlete has several short-term concerns:

- How badly am I hurt?
- Will I need surgery?
- How long will I be out?
- How much will this cost?

At this point, the examining physician's primary responsibilities are to make a preliminary diagnosis, consider other diagnostic possibilities, order needed tests, and develop an initial treatment plan. Other initial goals are to provide the injured athlete with the information needed to alleviate as much discomfort as possible, to confirm the diagnosis, to begin the injury treatment process, and to prepare the athlete for future decisions that must be made relative to the injury.

The physician must also address the psychological and emotional concerns of the injured athlete by providing some preliminary thoughts on the nature of the injury and some hope of shortly learning of the severity of the injury. Although the initial exam is often a significant source of doubt and worry, it can also offer information, perspective, and hope that can prepare the athlete to more positively handle the later stages of the injury management process.

NATURE OF ATHLETIC INJURIES

Sports injuries are different from most other injuries in that they usually involve strong, athletic, skilled individuals performing at a high level of activity. In the mind of most athletes, whether "weekend warriors" or seriously committed, the injury needs to be treated and rehabilitated quickly. Most athletes have a mind-set to do whatever is necessary to return to doing something that they love, rather than something they must do, and to return to their previous level of performance.

Understanding and customizing the care of each type of injured athlete is what this book is all about. "Weekend warriors" are highly motivated to return to their sport, but they often have other obligations that take priority and may affect their ability to approach rehabilitation with 100% commitment. In contrast, injured high-level athletes can devote their time and energy exclusively to their rehabilitation.

TYPES OF ATHLETIC INJURIES

There are generally three different types of athletic injuries: acute, chronic, and acute onset of a chronic condition. Acute injuries are most often fairly straightforward in that there was some injury mechanism—

either intrinsic (e.g., an athlete coming down from a spike in volleyball landed on an inverted ankle) or extrinsic (e.g., a soccer player injured a knee when slide tackled by an opponent). Determining the mechanism of injury, complete with limb and body position, often yields valuable clues as to the nature of the injury.

Chronic injuries may be a little more elusive then acute ones in that their history is oftentimes unclear. They may be of short duration (e.g., an athlete noticed that his shins started bothering him a week ago) or of much longer duration (e.g., complaints of lower back pain have come and gone for years). These too may be of intrinsic means (e.g., inherent biomechanical predisposition) or extrinsic means (e.g., change in footwear). Chronic injuries warrant further questioning about any other potential predisposing factors. Considerations such as previous similar injury, a new training surface or program, or introduction of a new sport-specific technique are a few examples of pertinent clues.

The third type of injury is acute onset of a chronic injury. These are the ankle sprains in the athlete with a grossly unstable ankle, shoulder dislocation of a shoulder that chronically subluxates, or disc herniation in the patient with chronic lower back pain. These injuries as well warrant more in-depth investigation into their history and previous treatment approaches.

The type of injury—acute, chronic, or acute-on-chronic—influences the mind-set of the patient. The acutely injured patient without a previous history of that particular injury generally is open-minded toward whatever diagnosis and treatment the physician offers. Meanwhile, the physician desires to, first, make an accurate diagnosis based on the history, examination, and any diagnostic studies such as an X ray or magnetic resonance imaging (MRI); then to convince the patient that the diagnosis is correct; and finally to develop a treatment plan that will be effective and timely. A follow-up schedule is created to confirm that the injury has been successfully treated and that the athlete has returned to a level better than that before the injury. Although these steps will hold true for acute, chronic, and acute-on-chronic injuries, the path to them varies depending on a host of factors.

The plight of the injured athlete occurs long before the athlete is seen in the physician's office. It occurs immediately at the time of the injury. How the athlete was initially treated when the injury occurred can have a lasting impact on the healing process—both physically and psychologically. The athlete's initial care may have been as comprehensive as having had a physician on-site to accurately diagnose and care for the athlete to having the athlete self-treat with significantly limited knowledge and resources.

INITIAL CARE OF THE ATHLETIC INJURY

When an injury occurs, it is essential that the proper initial treatment be administered. Regardless of whether medical supervision is carried out by the coach or by a trained sports medicine professional, a plan of action for when an injury occurs is critical for optimal care. An important component of such a plan is a referral base of qualified sports medicine professionals to whom athletes can readily turn. Athletes should not have to be responsible for finding proper care for an injury.

Wherever possible, a certified athletic trainer (ATC) should be present to provide initial care for injuries. The ATC's role is to perform preparatory tasks for injury prevention, athletic event coverage (including practices), rehabilitation services, and accurate injury assessment and treatment. The ATC is also responsible for coordinating efforts of the athlete, coach, and physician in designing the optimal treatment approach. When a trained professional is not present, athletes should seek out professional guidance as the injury warrants according to their level of pain and incapacitation.

After initial self-treatment or treatment by a trained professional, evaluation by a physician specializing in sports injuries may be required. These physicians have extensive experience in treating athletic injuries and typically work with the athlete to design a treatment approach that is more accommodating for active people. They understand the mind-set of the athlete and try to formulate the most aggressive care possible without compromising the injury itself. They also have considerable experience working with athletes, athletic trainers, and physical therapists in rehabilitating sports injuries, which is a critical factor for optimal outcomes.

THE EVALUATION PROCESS

The initial examination by the physician is a series of steps aimed at identifying the pathology of the injury and developing an appropriate treatment plan. Taking a detailed history, palpating, assessing active and passive range of motion, performing special manual tests, and ordering diagnostic tests (e.g., X rays and MRI) are the key tools that a physician uses to identify the specific nature of the injury.

The first step in the evaluation process is meeting the patient. Many physicians and patients do not fully appreciate the importance of this introduction to the overall injury management process. This initial contact sets the tone for the physician–patient relationship and can affect the efficacy of the treatment and rehabilitation plan. Although there are many ways to make an introduction, the messages are few. The patient wants to say, "This is me and my injury. Please take care of me." The doctor wants to say, "I am here to care for you, and I am interested in getting to know you too."

After initial introductions, we like to ask the patient what happened, along with the question, "What do *you* think you have done to yourself?" Although some patients do not like this question and respond with, "That's what I'm paying you to find out," most appreciate being asked for input and are often correct in their diagnosis.

The next step in the evaluation process is to take an accurate history, collecting all of the information related to the injury (see Figure 1.1). Examples of questions to ask include the following: How did the injury occur? Had there been previous problems with the area injured? Did the athlete hear a pop or snap at the time of injury? Was the athlete able to continue to participate in the sport? If the injury is a chronic one, were there any recent changes in equipment, setting, or schedule? An accurate history is important because it can often provide the diagnosis, eliminating the need for additional testing.

We recommend that the history be taken three times—first by the nurse practitioner, second by the orthopedic surgeon, and third by the rehabilitation professional. Although this may be somewhat annoying to some patients, each practitioner takes the history differently and asks different, yet relevant, questions. Also, patients often tell each practitioner of different concerns. Even though the events and the details may not change significantly, the different perspectives in the approaches to history taking provide valuable information in formulating a comprehensive diagnostic and treatment plan. Additionally, a patient's resisting this team approach to evaluation should raise red flags about the patient. Will the patient respond to a team approach? Is the patient going to be too demanding to effectively care for?

Once the history has been obtained, a comprehensive evaluation that involves observation, palpation, and muscle, gait, and neuromotor testing

HISTORY OF INJURY QUESTIONNAIRE

Name: _____

Occupation: _____

What is injured? _____

How and when were you injured? _____

_____

What were your symptoms?
Swelling ☐   Bruising ☐   Instability ☐   Pain ☐   Weakness ☐   Other ☐

_____

Did you hear a pop or snap?   Yes ☐   No ☐

Were you able to continue to participate following the injury? Yes ☐   No ☐

Have you seen other doctors for this injury?   Yes ☐   No ☐

Doctor's name and number: _____

Diagnosis given? _____

What treatment did you receive? _____

Did the treatment help?   Yes ☐   No ☐

What hurts now? _____

How does it feel now? _____

What can you not do? _____

What would you like to do? What are your goals?_____

_____

List all previous operations or significant illnesses and dates:_____

_____

List all medications you are taking: _____

_____

List any allergies you have to medication: _____

List special dietary habits, supplements: _____

_____

Do you belong to a gym?   Yes ☐   No ☐

Do you have access to a pool?   Yes ☐   No ☐

    Where? _____

(continues)

Figure 1.1. History of Injury Questionnaire.

Who referred you to this office?	Who is your family physician?
Name: _____	Name: _____
Address: _____	Address: _____
Phone: _____	Phone: _____

Figure 1.1. *Continued.*

is conducted. Figure 1.2 provides a sample evaluation form for a knee injury. Observation of swelling, redness, and skin condition provides some preliminary indications of the location and degree of trauma to the injured area. It also offers the physician guidance as to the type and intensity of palpation that should be employed.

Palpation is conducted to detect any subtle swelling, areas of marked temperature change, point tenderness, or abnormalities such as muscle defects or atrophy, as well as to determine muscle response. Most important, palpation is often the first manual contact the patient has with the physician. We recommend that the uninjured side be examined first, for example, the left knee if the right knee is the injured one. This gives the patient an opportunity to become familiar with how the doctor is going to touch the patient. The uninjured side can also serve as a model of what "normal" should feel like when the injured side is tested. Examining the uninjured side permits the doctor to look into the patient's eyes while a nonpainful test is being performed to assess the patient's confidence, mood, level of anxiety, and ability to communicate both verbally and nonverbally. This exam is a critical step in building trust between the physician and the patient. If examination of the uninjured side is uncomfortable for the patient, it is unlikely that the remainder of the physician–patient relationship will be comfortable.

In inspecting the injured area, carefully picking it up or holding it in a supportive way that does not elicit pain helps establish the patient's comfort and trust in the physical examination. Painful maneuvers should be saved until the end of the evaluation if possible. Whenever possible, the patient should be asked to move an injured joint through a range of motion while the physician supports the limb. This step further strengthens the patient's comfort and trust in the physician.

(*text continues on p. 15*)

INITIAL KNEE EVALUATION FORM

Name: _____ Date: _____

Who referred you? _____ Address: _____

Who is your internist? _____

Date of injury: _____ Injured knee: right ☐ left ☐

Chief complaint: _____

_____

What is your diagnosis? _____

History of incident: _____

_____

_____

_____

Any previous problems with this knee? No ☐ Yes ☐ _____

Have you ever had an X ray or MRI? No ☐ Yes ☐ _____

Have you ever had surgery on this knee? No ☐ Yes ☐ _____

Pain: Day +/− Night +/− Activity Related +/−

Where exactly? _____

Aggravating factors: _____

Alleviating factors: _____

Past medical history: _____

_____

Medications: _____

Allergies to medications: _____

Sports/activities participate in: _____

Sports/activities unable to participate in: _____

What is your goal?_____

Injured Knee

Pain: At Rest: None / Mild / Moderate / Severe

    With Activities: None / Mild / Moderate / Severe

    Swelling: None / Mild / Marked / Related to activity

(continues)

Figure 1.2. Initial Knee Evaluation Form. *Note.* ACL = anterior cruciate ligament; EHL = extensor hallucis longus; ITB = iliotibial bend; LCL = lateral collateral ligament; MCL = medial collateral ligament; MRI = magnetic resonance imaging; NSAID = nonsteroidal anti-inflammatory drug; PCL = posterior collateral ligament.

Giving Way: None / Sensation of Giving Way / Actual Giving Way

Locking: None / Sensation of Locking Way / Actual Locking

Ascending Stairs: Normal / With Difficulty / Cannot

Descending Stairs Normal / With Difficulty / Cannot

Measurements	Right	Left
Thigh girth (15 cm from proximal patella)	____	____
Thigh girth (5 cm from proximal patella)	____	____
Calf girth (10 cm from proximal patella)	____	____
Leg length Same Difference ___ cm Right or Left		

Range of Motion	Right	Left
1. X: flex	____	____
2. Y: O	____	____
3. Z: hypertension	____	____

KT Measurement	Right	Left
Actual Flexion Angle	____	____
Heel Position	____	____
Posterior		
15 pounds	____	____
20 pounds	____	____
Anterior		
15 pounds	____	____
20 pounds	____	____
30 pounds	____	____
Manual Maximum Displacement	____	____
Quadriceps Active Displacement	____	____

Inspection

Swelling: 0 1+ 2+ 3+ Scars: No ☐ Yes ☐ Where: _____

Baker's Cyst: No ☐ Yes ☐

(continues)

Figure 1.2. *Continued.*

Gait:	Normal	Limp	Unstable	Limp with Running	
	Posterior Lateral Corner Thrust				
Alignment:	Varus	Valgus	Neutral		

Palpation		Right	Left

Pain

	Right	Left
Quad Tendon	＿＿	＿＿
Medical Patella Facet	＿＿	＿＿
Lateral Patella Facet	＿＿	＿＿
Medial Retinaculum	＿＿	＿＿
Lateral Retinaculum	＿＿	＿＿
MCL, Femoral Insertion	＿＿	＿＿
MCL, Tibial Insertion	＿＿	＿＿
Joint Line Medial	＿＿	＿＿
Joint Line Lateral	＿＿	＿＿
Patellar Tendon	＿＿	＿＿
Tibial Tubercle	＿＿	＿＿
ITB	＿＿	＿＿
Pes Anserinus	＿＿	＿＿
Posterior Knee, Medial	＿＿	＿＿
Posterior Knee, Lateral	＿＿	＿＿

Crepitus

	Right	Left
Medial Patella Facet	＿＿	＿＿
Lateral Patella Facet	＿＿	＿＿
Trochlea	＿＿	＿＿
Joint Line Medial	＿＿	＿＿
Joint Line Lateral	＿＿	＿＿

Meniscus Tests

Medial Meniscus

	Right	Left
Apley's Pain	＿＿	＿＿
McMurray's Pop	＿＿	＿＿

(*continues*)

Figure 1.2. *Continued.*

Lateral Meniscus

    Apley's Pain   ____   ____

    McMurray's Pop   ____   ____

Laxity Test

	Left	Right
Medial Laxity	0 1+ 2+ 3+	0 1+ 2+ 3+
Lateral Laxity	0 1+ 2+ 3+	0 1+ 2+ 3+
Posterior Lateral Laxity	0 1+ 2+ 3+	0 1+ 2+ 3+
Posterior Medial Laxity	0 1+ 2+ 3+	0 1+ 2+ 3+
Lachman's	0 1+ 2+ 3+	0 1+ 2+ 3+
Anterior Drawer	0 1+ 2+ 3+	0 1+ 2+ 3+

Pivot Shift   0 Pivot Guide   1+ 2+ 3+
                 0 Pivot Guide   1+ 2+ 3+

	Left	Right
Reverse Pivot Shift	0 1+ 2+ 3+	0 1+ 2+ 3+
Posterior Drawer	0 1+ 2+ 3+	0 1+ 2+ 3+

Plica   Suprapatellar

    Medial   + / −   + / −   + / −   + / −

    Lateral   + / −   + / −   + / −   + / −

Motor Exam

	Right	Left
Quads	/5	/5
Hamstrings	/5	/5
Hip Flexors	/5	/5
Hip Adductors	/5	/5
Hip Abductors	/5	/5
Plantar Flexion	/5	/5
Dorsi Flexion	/5	/5
EHL	/5	/5
Ankle Inversion	/5	/5
Ankle Eversion	/5	/5

Review of X Ray   Negative   Dictation   None

                                                    (*continues*)

Figure 1.2. *Continued.*

MRI Reading	Negative	Chondral Lesion:
	Torn Meniscus (Medial / Lateral)	Med / Lat / Pat / Troc
	Torn ACL / PCL	Contusion
	Baker's Cyst	Effusion
	Other: _____	

Clinical Impression

ACL Tear / PCL Tear /MCL Tear / LCL Tear

Posterior Lateral Corner Instability

Baker's Cyst

ITB Tendinitis

Lateral Meniscus Tear / Medial Meniscus Tear

Patellar Arthritis

Patellar Subluxation / Dislocation

Patellar Tendinitis

Pes Anserinus Inflammation

Pes Planus

Plica

Synovitis

Post Traumatic Arthritis

Chondral Lesion

Other: _____

Further Work Up MRI / Bone Scan / Blood Work

Treatment Plan Exercise Training / Physical Therapy / Surgery

Brace / Cortisone / NSAIDs

Follow-Up Schedule:

Post MRI _____ / Weeks _____

Copy of Evaluation To:

Patient: _____

MD: _____

Other: _____

Figure 1.2. *Continued.*

Assessing the quality of active and passive motion is the next step in injury evaluation. If the athlete is fairly mobile and functional, then assessing active motion first can oftentimes reveal restrictions in passive motion. If there are restrictions in the active motion, then testing the passive motion of the joint can determine true pathology and restrictions. It is important when assessing the passive motion of the injured area that the amount of passive glide of the articulation be evaluated as well. For instance, if an athlete with shoulder pain has limited active range of motion into overhead positions and full passive motion into all planes, and the glide of the glenohumeral joint is restricted posteriorly and inferiorly, this is an important finding—indicating tight posterior capsule—that needs to be addressed during the rehabilitation process. Assessing any biomechanical problems, such as those exhibited during gait or when performing movement patterns, yields additional clues that help in designing the treatment approach.

Diagnostic tests need to be obtained to confirm many diagnoses. Whether X rays or MRIs, these tests have personal and financial risks, as well as diagnostic implications. Counseling patients about these concerns before the tests are ordered can relieve worry and stress that they may experience. The opportunity to review the results with the patient as soon as they are obtained diminishes the uncertainty and discomfort. Whenever possible, we recommend obtaining X rays and MRIs and reviewing the results on the day of the first visit. If this is not possible, we ask the patient to return to the office as soon as possible to review the results with the physician. The studies act as independent confirmation of the diagnosis and often eliminate the need for second opinions for many patients.

In addition to the objective assessments, functional evaluations are useful in identifying the practical limitations of the injury. This process helps both the sports medicine team and the injured athlete in clarifying the severity of the injury at a functional level. Two common evaluation instruments for this purpose are the International Knee Documentation Committee (IKDC) Subjective Knee Evaluation Form (American Orthopaedic Society for Sports Medicine, 1999; see Figure 1.3) and the Tegner Activity Level Scale (Tegner & Lysolm, 1985; see Figure 1.4).

Following the history, physical exam, and diagnostic studies, a consultation is conducted to synthesize the diverse data obtained from the patient. We suggest meeting with the patient in a room other than the examining room to discuss the findings and the treatment plan. This

(*text continues on p. 19*)

IKDC SUBJECTIVE KNEE EVALUATION FORM

Your Full Name _____

Today's Date ____ / ____ / ____   Date of Injury ____ / ____ / ____

SYMPTOMS:

1. What is the highest level of activity that you can perform without significant knee pain?

   ☐ Very strenuous activities like jumping or pivoting as in basketball or soccer
   ☐ Strenuous activities like heavy physical work, skiing or tennis
   ☐ Moderate activities like moderate physical work, running or jogging
   ☐ Light activities like walking, housework or yard work
   ☐ Unable to perform any of the above activities due to knee pain

2. During the past 4 weeks, or since your injury, how often have you had pain?

	0	1	2	3	4	5	6	7	8	9	10	
Never	☐	☐	☐	☐	☐	☐	☐	☐	☐	☐	☐	Constant

3. If you have pain, how severe is it?

	0	1	2	3	4	5	6	7	8	9	10	
No pain	☐	☐	☐	☐	☐	☐	☐	☐	☐	☐	☐	Worst pain imaginable

4. During the past 4 weeks, or since your injury, how stiff or swollen was your knee?

   ☐ Not at all   ☐ Mildly   ☐ Moderately   ☐ Very   ☐ Extremely

5. What is the highest level of activity you can perform without significant swelling in your knee?

   ☐ Very strenuous like jumping or pivoting as in basketball or soccer
   ☐ Strenuous activities like heavy physical work, skiing or tennis
   ☐ Moderate activities like moderate physical work, running or jogging
   ☐ Light activities like walking, housework or yard work
   ☐ Unable to perform any of the above activities due to knee swelling

6. During the past 4 weeks, or since your injury, did your knee lock or catch?

   ☐ Yes   ☐ No

(continues)

Figure 1.3. Functional Evaluation. *Note.* Adapted from *IKDC Subjective Knee Evaluation Form*, by American Orthopaedic Society for Sports Medicine, 1999, retrieved October 21, 2002, from http://aclstudygroup.com/IKDC%20form .htm#KDC%20SUBJECTIVE%20KNEE%20EVALUATION%20FORM

7. What is the highest level of activity you can perform without significant giving way in your knee?

   ☐ Very strenuous activities like jumping or pivoting as in basketball or soccer

   ☐ Strenuous activities like heavy physical work, skiing or tennis

   ☐ Moderate activities like moderate physical work, running or jogging

   ☐ Light activities like walking, housework or yard work

   ☐ Unable to perform any of the above activities due to giving way of the knee

SPORTS ACTIVITIES:

8. What is the highest level of activity you can participate in on a regular basis?

   ☐ Very strenuous activities like jumping or pivoting as in basketball or soccer

   ☐ Strenuous activities like heavy physical work, skiing or tennis

   ☐ Moderate activities like moderate physical work, running or jogging

   ☐ Light activities like walking, housework or yard work

   ☐ Unable to perform any of the above activities due to knee pain

9. How does your knee affect your ability to:

	Not difficult at all	Minimally difficult	Moderately difficult	Extremely difficult	Unable to do
a. Go up stairs	☐	☐	☐	☐	☐
b. Go down stairs	☐	☐	☐	☐	☐
c. Kneel on the front of your knee	☐	☐	☐	☐	☐
d. Squat	☐	☐	☐	☐	☐
e. Sit with your knee bent	☐	☐	☐	☐	☐
f. Rise from a chair	☐	☐	☐	☐	☐
g. Run straight ahead	☐	☐	☐	☐	☐
h. Jump and land on your involved leg	☐	☐	☐	☐	☐
i. Stop and start quickly	☐	☐	☐	☐	☐

(continues)

Figure 1.3. *Continued.*

TEGNER ACTIVITY LEVEL SCALE

Please indicate in the spaces below the HIGHEST level of activity that you participated in <u>BEFORE YOUR INJURY</u> and the highest level you are able to participate in <u>CURRENTLY.</u>

Level 10	Competitive sports: soccer, football, rugby (national elite)
Level 9	Competitive sports: soccer, football, rugby (lower divisions), ice hockey, wrestling, gymnastics, basketball
Level 8	Competitive sports: racquetball or bandy, squash or badminton, track and field athletics (jumping, etc.), down-hill skiing
Level 7	Competitive sports: tennis, running, motorcars speed-way, handball Recreational sports: soccer, football, rugby, bandy, ice hockey, basketball, squash, racquetball, running
Level 6	Recreational sports: tennis and badminton, handball, racquetball, downhill skiing, jogging at least 5 times per week
Level 5	Work-heavy labor (construction, etc.) Competitive sports: cycling, cross-country skiing Recreational sports: jogging on uneven ground at least twice weekly
Level 4	Work: moderately heavy labor (e.g., truck driving)
Level 3	Work: light labor (nursing, etc.)
Level 2	Work: light labor Walking on uneven ground possible, but impossible to backpack or hike
Level 1	Work: sedentary (secretarial, etc.)
Level 0	Sick leave or disability pension because of knee problems
BEFORE INJURY: Level _____	CURRENT: Level _____

Figure 1.4. Tegner Activity Level Scale. *Note.* From "Rating Systems in the Evaluation of Knee Ligament Injuries," by Y. Tegner and J. Lysholm, 1985, *Clinical Orthopaedics and Related Research, 198,* pp. 43–49. Copyright 1985 by Lippincott, Williams & Wilkins. Reprinted with permission.

begin immediately. The patient should meet with the physical therapist and athletic trainer, in addition to a sports nutritionist and massage therapist if indicated. The rehabilitation program is designed at that point, and a follow-up schedule of treatment is agreed upon. If surgery is necessary, a presurgical training program is devised to keep the patient exercising around the injured area. The rehabilitation staff helps to develop a physical conditioning program around the injured area to ensure that overall fitness is not compromised. For example, a patient with a knee injury can usually ride a stationary bicycle to train the uninjured leg while the injured leg rests on a chair. These efforts immediately convey to the patient that the injury will not inhibit him or her from continuing to grow as an athlete. It also instills a strong sense of hope in the very earliest stages of the athlete's rehabilitation.

PSYCHOLOGICAL AND EMOTIONAL CONCERNS IMMEDIATELY FOLLOWING INJURY

An injury to athletes is, at best, an irritating "bump in the road" and, at worst, a traumatic experience that can have significant negative ramifications in their lives. Common reactions include shock, denial, unrealistic expectations of recovery, depression, and stress (Heil, 1993). The degree of difficulty that athletes have in response to an injury depends largely on its severity and its treatment implications in terms of pain, effort, time required for rehabilitation, and physical limitations.

Before any of these issues are addressed, the immediate implications of the injury must be considered. A serious injury can have a powerful impact on many aspects of an athlete's life. The most obvious effect is that it will substantially alter the person's ability to engage in his or her sport. One might think that this would be most important for athletes who perform at the professional and world-class levels, because their livelihoods depend on their sports participation. However, we have found that the level of athletic involvement is less important than the "investment" that athletes have in their athletic lives. Although not at a financial level, "weekend warriors" who are highly invested in their sports can have an equally strong reaction to an injury as an accomplished athlete. It is this investment that can cause additional difficulties in other parts of athletes' lives.

The notion of investment in sports participation is related to the degree to which a person's self-identity—how one perceives oneself—depends on athletic pursuits. For those whose athletic identity composes a large part of their overall self-identity, removal of the sport due to injury will influence them greatly. Research suggests that there is a significant relationship between athletic identity and severity of psychological and emotional difficulties in response to an injury (Brewer, 1993). Questions like "Who am I?" and "What do I do now?" are common reactions of injured athletes who are highly invested in their sport.

An injury can also affect athletes socially. If their primary social system—friends, acquaintances, activities—revolves around their sport, an injury can isolate them from needed support and exacerbate their emotional difficulties. The injury can also create a void in how they fill their time and how they gain enjoyment and satisfaction. As a result, athletes experience boredom, which can feed into more significant emotional difficulties.

The probability of psychological problems depends on the severity of the injury. Athletes who sustain a minor injury, such as a second-degree sprain, might have a transitory negative reaction immediately after the injury, particularly prior to an accurate diagnosis or if it keeps them from participating in an important competition. However, these responses are typically short-lived as soon as it becomes clear that the injury is not serious and will not involve a prolonged duration away from their sport. Consequently, less vigilance for psychological distress is required for athletes who suffer a minor injury.

Psychological problems are most common among athletes who have experienced a serious injury requiring a lengthy and potentially painful rehabilitation (Heil, 1993), because the pain is usually more significant, returning to sports participation will take longer, rehabilitation will be protracted and difficult, and concerns about a full recovery will be prominent. The probability of psychological distress is high among athletes with serious injury, and close attention should be paid to negative reactions during the entire injury management process.

Immediately following an injury, athletes' focus is in the past, on the injury itself. There is often a sense of confusion ("What happened?"), self-examination ("Why me?"), and loss ("What am I going to do?"). The sooner injured athletes can shift their focus away from the past, the negative, and the uncontrollable and onto the present, the positive, and the controllable, the more comfortable they will feel and the fewer psychological difficulties they will experience.

Although negative reactions to injury can emerge at any time in the recovery process, they are most likely to emerge at several specific points during injury management (Heil, 1993). One of the points is immediately after the injury and prior to diagnosis (see Table 1.1). The unpredictability of the injury, the pain experienced, and the uncertainty of the future can all combine to create a powerful, and usually negative, emotional reaction. Healthy adaptation is likely to occur as the athlete comes to accept the injury, recognizes the inevitability of what may lie ahead, gains a better understanding of and familiarity with the injury management process, and receives adequate social support to attenuate the negative emotions.

TABLE 1.1
Likely Points of Psychological Problems
During Rehabilitation

Point of Rehabilitation	Causes of Psychological Distress	Contributors to Adaptation
Immediately Postinjury	Suddenness of injury	Acceptance of injury
	Lack of familiarity, predictability, control	Recognition of inevitability of injury
	Disruption of goals	Social support
	Pain and discomfort	
	Uncertainty of future	
Following Diagnosis	Realization of severity of injury	Understanding of meaning of diagnosis
	Recognition of courses of rehabilitation	Shift to constructive, future orientation
	Sense of hopelessness in facing recovery	Education about rehabilitation process
	Doubts about complete recovery	Examples of injured athletes who recovered
If Surgery Is Required	Realization of seriousness of injury	Understanding the benefits of surgery
	Unfamiliarity with surgery	Education about the surgery process
	Impact of surgery on future participation	Successful repair of the injury

(continues)

TABLE 1.1. *Continued.*

Point of Rehabilitation	Causes of Psychological Distress	Contributors to Adaptation
Third Quarter of Rehabilitation Period	Physically tired	Focus on positive aspects of rehabilitation
	Emotionally drained	
	Depleted resources for remainder of recovery	Obtain adequate rest
		Experience successes during rehabilitation
	Frustration over length of rehabilitation	See progress toward complete recovery
Approaching Return to Sport	Awareness of time and effort invested	Focus on quality of rehabilitation
	Facing possibility of failure	Recognize readiness for return to sport
		Recall the time and effort that was put in
		Focus on desire to return to sport

Note. From *Psychological Approaches to Sports Injury Rehabilitation* (p. 67), by J. Taylor and S. Taylor, 1997, Austin, TX: PRO-ED. Copyright 1997 by PRO-ED, Inc. Reprinted with permission.

CHAPTER 2

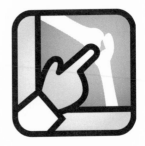

Diagnosis and Treatment

Often, athletes do not fully understand how they got hurt. They know the situation in which it occurred, but most athletic injuries happen in a training or competitive situation like ones in which the athlete has performed many times. A big question, then, for injured athletes is, Why did I get injured this time? Was the injury a freak accident that is unlikely to happen again, or did I do something that precipitated the injury? The answer to this question has a powerfully relieving effect. If the accident was a freak occurrence, then the athlete can feel more comfortable that it is not likely to happen again. If the athlete did something to cause the injury, then he or she can understand how not to let it happen again, thus providing a sense of control over the injury. The examining physician can help the athlete answer this question by connecting the nature of the injury, as determined by the diagnosis, to the actions that led to the injury.

The next question that needs to be answered is, Was the preliminary intervention helpful? The answer to this question provides the injured athlete with some sense of the severity of the injury. If the injury responded well to the initial treatment, then perhaps it is not that serious. The efficacy of the initial treatment will also guide the physician in making a diagnosis. Injured athletes always hope their injury is not serious and will look to the preliminary treatment as some evidence in support of this optimism, so learning that the treatment was not effective can be traumatic to an injured athlete. Therefore, the physician must be especially sensitive about how this information is communicated.

With these past-oriented questions answered, the injured athlete can now focus on the present. This is the point at which the athlete gains a full understanding and appreciation of the severity of the injury. This shift in focus creates additional concern, raising more questions about the injury: What do the test results show? What is the specific diagnosis of the injury?

The answers to these questions relieve uncertainty about the seriousness of the injury by making clear the precise nature of the injury. There is tremendous relief if the injury is not as serious as anticipated and increased doubt and stress if the injury is more severe than expected. Regardless of how serious the injury is, at least the athlete knows where he or she stands.

PATIENT REACTIONS

If the injury is severe, psychological distress may be evident following diagnosis when the magnitude of the injury and the length and difficulty of rehabilitation become clear. Adaptation usually results as the athlete gains a better understanding of the injury, becomes more familiar with the impending rehabilitation, is better able to predict events, and develops a greater sense of control over the rehabilitation. If the injury requires surgery, psychological difficulties may arise from the often unexpected seriousness of the injury and from concerns about the surgical experience and the ramifications of surgery on future sports participation. Adaptation is likely to occur with understanding of the benefits of surgery to recovery, education about the surgery process, and successful repair of the injury. Physicians and other members of the sports medicine team should be sensitive to patient reactions to their diagnosis and respond in a proactive and positive manner.

CONFIRMATION OF DIAGNOSIS

At this point, the injured athlete's main focus is on what has happened and what can be done to fix it. After acute injuries, athletes may replay the occurrence of injury. Those injuries that were sustained by outside forces (e.g., a soccer slide tackle) are sometimes easier to handle mentally than those caused by intrinsic means (e.g., landing awkwardly on the knee). More elusive are the chronic injuries for which the athlete cannot determine any predisposing factors.

The intrinsic type of injury can sometimes be caused by secondary means. That is, the activity precipitated the injury, but secondary factors led to the symptoms. For instance, an athlete who has been compensating for a previous ankle injury may cause a back condition due to the change in mechanics, or an athlete develops tendinitis of the knee as a result of significant restrictions in hip and pelvis mobility. These preventable types of injuries need to be treated physically in such a way as to address underlying pathology and psychologically so as not to make the athlete feel responsible or guilty for not having prevented them. Therefore, the initial examination must be as thorough as possible. As discussed in Chapter 1, taking a comprehensive history, performing all appropriate tests, assessing gait and biomechanics, and developing a working diagnosis to institute treatment are the key elements. Treatment should be initiated as soon as possible so that the athlete does not have any "down time" in recuperating from the injury. Providing a detailed explanation of the treatment approach empowers the patient. It is one of the few things over which the injured athlete actually has control. Communicating this information to all members of the sports medicine team will also aid in keeping consistency, not only in the treatment approach but also in what the athlete is told.

Conducting a thorough initial examination and maintaining consistency in communications bear on the two most important components in the treatment of athletic injuries—accuracy of the working diagnosis (including all predisposing factors) and trust of the athlete in the sports medicine team. The first component is critical because it is the driving force behind the treatment approach. Incorrect, inadequate, or inconclusive diagnoses will have a deleterious effect on the ultimate outcome of the injury. In the fifth century B.C., Hippocrates wrote, "first, do no harm" (Clayman, 1989). Health care providers must make it their utmost priority to do nothing that might cause harm to a patient. If there is any doubt as to the accuracy of the diagnosis or the judiciousness of the treatment plan, they should be reconsidered, often by conducting follow-up exams or tests or referring to a specialist.

The athlete must appreciate that the sports medicine team knows and understands him or her and that they have a thorough understanding of the injuries and subsequent trauma. This trust can be fostered with an understanding of the sport in which the injured athlete participates and what is needed for the athlete to return to the sport. This knowledge can be gained in several ways. It can be learned through active participation in the sport by a member of the sports medicine team. This understanding can be obtained through the experience of members of the sports medicine team in previous treatment of other athletes in the sport. If the sport is esoteric enough, a member of the sports medicine team can do a brief study of the sport to learn about its unique demands relative to injured athletes.

FOLLOW-UP TREATMENT PLAN

After the initial assessment and initiation of treatment, we recommend a plan of care that could be deemed "conservative-aggressive." *Conservative* implies that all nonsurgical options will be investigated and any that are instituted will not compromise the ultimate treatment outcome. (Some conditions require urgent surgical intervention, and these are addressed in later chapters.) *Conservative* also denotes restricting activity and deleterious forces on the healing structures in the early stages to allow the athlete to get better faster and more comfortably. Some examples of this approach are restricting weight bearing for a severe ankle sprain and blocking the range of motion for a healing medial collateral ligament sprain in the knee. In both examples, the athlete would be able to return to sport no matter how the injury was handled in the early stages. Yet, the athlete would most probably end up with chronic instability, weakness, and increased susceptibility to reinjury. Proper care would allow the athlete to return in optimal condition with increased joint stability.

Aggressive entails using all appropriate treatment options together in the early stages and slowly eliminating treatment approaches that cease to be useful in promoting the patient's recovery. Proper assessment and ongoing evaluation of the patient by the sports medicine team help determine when certain treatment approaches are no longer considered necessary. For example, if an athlete has a diagnosis of shoulder impingement, the initial plan of care should entail anti-inflammatory medication and icing to reduce irritation, soft tissue and joint mobilization to improve shoulder function, flexibility and strengthening exercises to address imbalances, correction of postural and biomechanical flaws that might have contributed to the injury, and possibly even massage therapy and acupuncture to aid in reducing the symptoms associated with such a condition. Once the success of the initial intervention can be assessed, then the first items to be discontinued in the plan of care are the anti-inflammatory medications and the pain control techniques (massage therapy and acupuncture). Once the joint restrictions are worked out, then manual therapy and joint mobilization can be replaced by an individual home program for the athlete to return to a stronger level than before the injury.

Specialist Referrals

The field of sports medicine has changed dramatically over the past 20 years. The advent of new technologies, specialist physicians, and treatment approaches that advocate early mobilization have allowed athletes to return to their sport faster and stronger than ever. Athletic trainers have become more of a mainstay in the athletic arena, and physical therapists now have an orthopedic sports physical therapy division.

It used to be that when an athlete was injured, the athlete would be seen by the family physician and either treated directly or sent to an orthopedist if the situation warranted. Today athletes frequently go directly to their sports orthopedic surgeon. Sports orthopedic surgeons often specialize in shoulders, knees, foot and ankle injuries, dance injuries, and even sport-specific injuries. This move toward specialization has emphasized the importance of referral to appropriate specialists. In addition, the orthopedic physician may not be the doctor who will perform surgery, but rather provides the most comprehensive evaluation of the injury and directs patients to the most appropriate care.

Input from a neurologist, for instance, in the case of a football player with radicular symptoms is critical in deciding whether there are true cervical lesions or the problem is simply a case of residual "burners." In the case of Lisfranc fracture of the foot, appropriate referral would be to a foot and ankle specialist. This could mean the difference between return to full sports participation within a year or long-term residual dysfunction of the midfoot if the complex surgical procedure was performed incorrectly.

Additional Testing

There also exists the possibility of systemic conditions being masked as an orthopedic problem. An athlete presenting to an orthopedist with symptoms of chronic knee pain could be suffering from anything as straightforward as tendinitis or overuse trauma to more insidious problems such as osteomyolitis or reflex sympathetic dystrophy. This is a case where a thorough history, comprehensive clinical examination, and appropriate referral for additional tests are essential.

Several factors should be considered when analyzing tests results. First, clinical presentation must confirm or refute findings of any special test— an abnormal finding from magnetic resonance imaging (MRI) may not necessarily correlate with true pathology. For instance, if an athlete with lateral epicondylitis has an MRI that shows a ganglionic cyst in the medial musculature but not in the area where the athlete is having symptoms, then it can be assumed that the cyst is not problematic. Second, the quality of the reading by the reviewing party is essential to accurate diagnosis. A radiologist who does not specialize in joint injuries might provide a general reading of a joint MRI that misses important, subtle findings. We recommend that the orthopedic surgeon independently read all studies with the patient present and then compare that reading to the one obtained from the radiologist. We always provide our radiologists with a copy of the operative reports when the findings differ from what they had predicted. Any further workup requires that the athlete be put through some physical and financial inconvenience, and it is important that the physician be able to effectively utilize this information so that the patient does not think that it was all in vain. Even if the test results came back negative, assuring the patient that this is pertinent information that will allow the rehabilitation to proceed is helpful.

Therefore, it is important that the approach to reviewing test results with patients be consistent and diminish the chances of misinterpretation. Reviewing test results over the phone with a patient precludes a follow-up clinical examination or the opportunity to discuss in person the findings and subsequent treatment plan. The patient may feel overwhelmed when faced with the magnitude and ramifications of the injury, and a lot of things are going through the patient's mind during confirmation of the diagnosis. Hence, it is better for the patient to be able to see the images, watch the physician actually review the tests, be reexamined, and sit down with the physician to work together on a plan of care. This is beneficial for both the physician and the patient because they are able to assess the patient's response and discuss any potential alternatives immediately.

PHYSICIAN SELECTION

It is important for the injured athlete to feel that the physician selected to orchestrate his or her care can best guide the athlete to the most successful outcome possible. The following questions can assist the athlete in choosing a treating physician:

- What credentials, certifications, and qualifications does the physician have that would make him or her the best physician to treat me (e.g., is the physician fellowship trained in this field)?

- How many similar cases has the physician treated, and what was the success rate with these cases?

- From whom could I get a second opinion?

- Has the doctor written anything on the procedure, or can he or she provide anything written by others about the procedure?

- Would the physician undergo this procedure or recommend it for a family member?

- What does the office look like? Do I want to receive care there?

- Does the physician have a qualified and friendly office staff to assist in recovery?

- Does the physician appear kind and genuine?

- Do I feel comfortable asking the physician questions, and does the physician answer fully or evasively?

Because injured athletes are often not informed consumers, it is incumbent on the sports medicine professional who initially treats an athlete to offer these relevant questions and to assist the athlete in obtaining answers to guide him or her to the most qualified physician for the treatment of the injury.

The most common way in which patients find a physician and determine the physician's qualifications is through referral from a trusted primary care physician or a friend who has seen the physician for similar injuries. These word-of-mouth referrals have two benefits. They are expeditious for the injured athlete at a time when he or she is in pain and highly motivated to seek treatment. Second, these referrals are generally trusted by patients because they have faith in the person making the referral.

The Internet has also provided easy access to a wealth of information for judging physician qualifications. Online information from physicians' own Web sites and those of independent medical boards and professional associations can help injured athletes readily learn about what makes a physician qualified to treat their injury and which physicians meet those criteria. In addition, injured athletes can educate themselves about the nature of their injury and what the most appropriate courses of action are. All of these steps act to turn injured athletes into informed consumers in their search for a physician who can best treat their injury.

Because of the Internet, patients are better informed, with access to far more health information than ever before. However, too much information combined with no medical experience can be confusing and overwhelming to patients. Patients who demonstrate knowledge without the appropriate perspective and understanding can be somewhat off-putting to the physician. The sports medicine team should assess the degree of knowledge that a patient has and use it as an opportunity to clarify misconceptions, further educate the patient, and guide the patient to what is useful, reliable, and accurate.

Injured athletes can also rely on the physicians' own answers and their demeanor to assist them in selecting the physician to treat them. Along with the answers to the questions posed earlier, the sense of comfort and trust that an injured athlete feels with a physician should be a significant determinant in the selection process.

Three components are essential for building a trusting physician–patient relationship. First, physicians who are responsive to the physical, psychological, and emotional needs of their patients are going to foster confidence in the injured athletes. Second, physicians can provide injured athletes with clear and understandable information in response to the questions that they pose (or the physician poses on their behalf), like the ones listed earlier. Third, physicians must have confidence in their answers. Because most injured athletes are not familiar with the medical aspects of their injury or possible treatment options, they have no basis for having confidence in their own judgments. They look to their physician for that "vicarious" confidence. Physicians who are confident in their prescriptions, responsive to the "whole person" needs of their patients, and able to provide unambiguous information about the injury and possible courses of treatment will engender confidence and trust and will, most likely, provide effective treatment.

Injured athletes can also explore the physicians' qualifications. They can ask physicians to put them in touch with patients with a similar injury who were given a similar treatment plan. This direct feedback from someone who has shared the patient's experience can be a powerful source of comfort and confidence in a physician.

TREATMENT OPTIONS

Although the injured athlete now knows the seriousness of the injury, there is still, as in each step of the injury management process, continued uncertainty. The new source of concern is how the injury will be treated. The pertinent questions that the athlete must ask are

- What are my treatment options?
- How successful are these possible treatments?
- Which treatment should I select?

These questions lay the foundation for the critical decision making that will determine the course of treatment and recovery. Although it is the responsibility of the physician to provide the best care possible for the patient, the degree of information that each patient wants varies widely. The physician is responsible for determining the amount of information that will allow the patient to make an informed and comfortable decision about which treatment option to choose.

The physician must be sensitive to the importance of this decision to an injured athlete. Because treatment options are usually discussed immediately following confirmation of the diagnosis, the athlete may be experiencing some informational and emotional overload. The athlete is still trying to assimilate the meaning of the diagnosis within the context of his or her life, particularly if the injury is serious and will have significant impact. This context includes physical, social, financial, and daily functioning. In addition, the injury and, if the injury is serious, the rehabilitation that lies ahead, may trigger a rush of emotions, including frustration, anger, and despair.

The way in which the physician communicates the treatment options will have one of two effects. It will either add to the information overload and deepen the negative emotions the injured athlete is experiencing, or it will assist the injured athlete in integrating the diagnostic and treatment information and replace the negative affect with positive emotions and a sense of hope. This point in the injury management process is crucial because it is where the patient makes the transition from injured athlete to healing athlete. The attitude that the athlete takes out of this meeting often sets the tone for his or her immediate response to the diagnosis and treatment and can also have a long-term impact on the course and quality of rehabilitation and return to sport.

To create a positive framework for discussion of the treatment options, the physician should stress the likelihood of positive outcomes. Using the physician's experience, medical research, and examples of patients who have had similar injuries with successful recoveries can have a powerful buoying effect on the patient. The onus for a positive treatment should also be placed as much as possible on the athlete, thereby giving the athlete a greater sense of ownership and responsibility for his or her treatment and rehabilitation.

Selecting a Treatment Option

Developing an effective treatment approach entails careful thought and planning. The physician has a multitude of treatment options available to address even the most complicated cases. The physician chooses which options to present and to use based on a combination of the physician's impressions of the patient and the physician's experience. To arrive at those choices, input from each member of the sports medicine team who comes into contact with the patient is essential.

In addition, the treatment plan developed must meet not only the patient's physical needs, but also the patient's psychological and emotional capabilities. For example, intimidated, shy, or fearful patients may not respond to an advanced, complicated treatment plan. Conversely, a highly demanding patient with no interest in listening to anyone in the office other than the physician might not succeed in a program that involves a team approach. The dynamics between the patient, the physician, and the sports medicine team strongly influence the treatment options as well as the outcome.

Most physicians present treatment options in a biased manner. It is important to understand the doctor's bias. The physician should tell the patient of that bias and the rationale behind it. For example, when a patient presents with a torn meniscus cartilage, one orthopedic surgeon might emphasize the possibility of surgical repair of that torn cartilage. This treatment direction reflects the surgeon's 20 years of meniscus cartilage research and a strong belief that it is better to try to save the meniscus cartilage than to remove it. The benefits and risks are also described. In contrast, another surgeon might recommend removal of part of the meniscus cartilage and provide an equally compelling argument for this approach.

The patient may have a treatment bias as well. An injured athlete might tell the surgeon, "This is the middle of my professional career. I do not want any down time and want to avoid the risk of another surgery at this time." This patient's bias would argue against a meniscus repair. This physician–patient communication about treatment options also influences the risks the surgeon is willing to take, the time the clinic team is willing to spend with the patient, and the quality of the entire diagnostic and treatment experience.

How does the patient choose from among the treatment options presented? It depends on the confidence the patient has in the physician. If patients have confidence in their physician, then it is likely that they will have faith in the recommended treatment plan. The key to this trust is based on two things. First, the physician must be highly qualified to treat the patient's particular injury (see Chapter 4). Second, the patient must feel comfortable with the physician both professionally and personally and with how the physician communicates the diagnosis and treatment options. If the patient has confidence in the physician's qualifications to treat the injury and feels comfortable in the relationship, deciding on a treatment option will be easier. If the physician presents the information clearly and makes a definitive recommendation with a compelling argument to support it, and the physician would undergo the same treatment or recommend it for a family member, then, most often, the patient will choose that approach.

Developing a Treatment Plan

Guiding patients toward a successful outcome should be the approach taken in designing a treatment plan. Suboptimal outcomes can easily occur when patients fail to comply fully with the chosen course of treatment. This noncompliance may include not following treatment instructions, missing scheduled rehabilitation sessions, not performing home exercises, and not completing the full treatment and rehabilitation regimen. In developing a treatment plan, the patient and the physician must fashion one that the patient can expect to complete. To do so, it is essential that patients share their goals and expectations related to their chosen treatment and their return to sport.

Once selected, the treatment plan must be committed to fully to ensure a positive outcome. The commitment is a decision the patient must make in light of other life demands (e.g., work, family). Discussing with the physician those demands and the sacrifices they entail is often helpful. However, many patients feel uncomfortable about burdening the doctor with their personal situations. Often, however, they will speak about these concerns with other members of the sports medicine team, such as the nurse practitioner or the physical therapist. Someone on the team must ensure that these issues are addressed in a constructive way to enhance the probability of full commitment to the treatment plan and thus a positive outcome.

Educating the patient about the treatment approach is another critical part of the overall treatment plan. If the patient does not fully understand the ramifications of the treatment plan, then the sports medicine team would be unrealistic in expecting the patient to take an active role in the treatment process. Careful description of the damage caused by the injury and what can be done to remedy the situation is essential.

A scheduled plan of care—replete with short- and long-term goals—needs to be developed to ensure a positive response to treatment, determine the desired overall outcomes, and encourage patient participation. The overall treatment plan is outlined and supervised by the physician, who refers the patient to the appropriate rehabilitation professional for the various aspects of care (see the sample treatment plans in Tables 2.1 and 2.2).

In referring patients to associated health care providers, the physician should consider all available treatment options. Recognizing what each approach has to offer gives the physician more options for delivering optimal care. It is also always better to send a patient a little out of the way for treatment with a practitioner whose work is known and trusted than to risk the patient's receiving suboptimal care.

Although the nonsurgical treatment plan is established by the physician as an overview, rehabilitation professionals have their own set of goals for each patient. Consider, for example, an athlete given a diagnosis by the physician of lower back strain secondary to overuse. During the examination, the physician recognizes that the athlete has significant inflexibilities in the hip and pelvis. The physician's treatment plan might entail some form of anti-inflammatory medication, referral to a physical therapist or athletic trainer for soft tissue work and a flexibility program, and possibly another form of active, independent stretching, such as yoga or tai chi. The physical therapist or athletic trainer then evaluates the athlete and develops

(*text continues on p. 41*)

TABLE 2.1
Articular Cartilage Transplantation Treatment Plan

Surgical Procedure

- The procedure of articular cartilage transplantation is the treatment of articular cartilage defects or arthritis.
- The arthroscope is inserted and the structures of the knee joint are evaluated.
- The base of the defect is microfractured to stimulate a bleeding bed and healing response.
- An articular cartilage and cancellous bone plug is then harvested from the inter-condylar notch (a non–weight-bearing portion of the knee) and smashed into a paste.
- The paste is then impacted into the prepared defect to provide a matrix for new cartilage growth.

General Considerations

- Non–weight-bearing status for 4 weeks postop (resting foot on floor and driving are okay).
- Patient may be in a hinged brace for support and to serve as a reminder not to weight-bear. May wear unloading brace once swelling is down enough for proper fit.
- Push for full hyperextension equal to opposite side.
- Regular manual treatment should be conducted to the patella and all incisions—with particular attention to the anterior medial portal—to decrease the incidence of fibrosis.
- Light- to no-resistance stationary cycling is okay at 2 weeks postop.
- Early recruitment of the vastus medialis muscle is important.
- No resisted leg extension machines (isotonic or isokinetic) at any point.
- Low-impact activities for 3 months postop.

Use of the CPM for 6 hours a day for 4 weeks is imperative.

Week 1

- M.D. visit Day 1 postop to change dressing and review home program.
- Icing and elevation frequently per instruction.
- CPM at home for 6 hours daily/at night.
- Straight leg raise exercises (lying, seated, and standing), quadricep/ adductor/ gluteal sets, passive and active range-of-motion exercises.
- Hip and foot/ankle exercises, well-leg stationary cycling, upper-body conditioning.
- Pool/deep-water workouts after the first week.
- Soft tissue treatments and gentle mobilization to posterior musculature and patella.

(continues)

TABLE 2.1. *Continued.*

Week 1 *Continued.*

- Twice per day: sit at edge of bed and allow knee to bend to 90° or less for 1–2 minutes. Should feel a stretch with mild discomfort, but not sharp pain.
- Knee extension range of motion should be full.

Weeks 2–4

- M.D. visit at 5–10 days for suture removal (if any) and checkup.
- Manual resistance (proprioceptive neuromuscular facilitation [PNF] patterns) of the foot, ankle, and hip; core stabilization.
- Continue with pain control, range of motion, soft tissue treatments, and exercises.
- Non–weight-bearing aerobic exercises (e.g., unilateral cycling, Upper Body Ergometer [UBE], Schwinn Air-Dyne arms only).
- After 2 weeks, bilateral cycling with light to no resistance. Low spin cadence.

Weeks 5–6

- M.D. visit at 4 weeks postop, will progress to full weight bearing, weaning down to one crutch, cane, or no assistive device.
- Incorporate functional exercises (e.g., squats, lunges, shuttle/leg press, calf raises, step-ups/lateral step-ups).
- Balance/proprioception exercises.
- Road cycling as tolerated.
- Slow to rapid walking on treadmill (preferably a low-impact treadmill).
- Seek knee flexion range of motion.

Weeks 7–8

- Increase the intensity of functional exercises (e.g., add stretch cord for resistance, increase weight with weight lifting machines).
- Add lateral training exercises (side-stepping, Theraband resisted side-stepping).
- Patients should be walking without a limp and have full range of motion.

Weeks 9–12

- Low-impact activities until 12 weeks.
- Patients should be pursuing a home program with emphasis on sport/activity-specific training.

Note. From *Psychological Approaches to Sports Injury Rehabilitation* (p. 67), by J. Taylor and S. Taylor, 1997, Austin, TX: PRO-ED. Copyright 1997 by PRO-ED, Inc. Reprinted with permission.

TABLE 2.2
Inferior Glenohumeral Ligament Repair Treatment Plan

Surgical Procedure

- This procedure done to anchor or reattach the labrum to the glenoid.
- The procedure can be done arthroscopically or through an open incision.
- Our procedure is done arthroscopically with sutures taken through the torn labrum.
- One end of the suture is threaded through an anchor, which is embedded in the glenoid.
- The labrum is secured to the glenoid and anchor with arthroscopic slipknots.

General Considerations

- Use of a sling for 4 weeks postop unless otherwise indicated.
- Okay to shower once dressings are changed (Day 1).
- *Arm is restricted from these movements for 4 weeks:*
    Extension (backward) past the plane of the body
    External rotation (arm rotation outward) greater than 0° (straight in front); extensive repairs may require more restrictions
    For posterior repairs, avoid any internal rotation (turning in) past the body
- No passive forceful stretching into external rotation/extension for 3 months following an anterior repair or into internal rotation for a posterior repair.
- Maintenance of good postural positioning when performing all exercises.
- Aerobic conditioning throughout the rehabilitation process.
- M.D. follow-ups Day 1, Days 8–10, 1 month, 4 months, 6 months, and 1 year.
- All active exercises should be carefully monitored to minimize substitution or compensation.

Week 1 Postop

- M.D. office visit (Day 1) to change dressings and review home exercise program.
- Home program to consist of the following:
    Icing shoulder as often as able for the first 3–5 days
    Elbow flexion/extension, wrist and forearm strengthening, cervical stretches, postural education and exercises.
    Stationary bike, stair machine, and VersaClimber without putting weight on arms.

Weeks 2–4

- Pain control (e.g., cryotherapy, massage, electric stim).
- Begin isometrics in all planes as tolerated.
- Soft tissue treatments to scars and surrounding musculature.
- General conditioning as tolerated (include trunk flexion and extension exercises).

(continues)

TABLE 2.2. *Continued.*

Weeks 5–6

- Resting pain should be notably diminishing.
- Passive and active assisted range of motion (AAROM) flexion out to the scapular plane as tolerated (cane exercises, wall walking, table slide).
- Progress to active exercises from flexion into the scapular plane against gravity as tolerated.
  No resistance until able to perform 30 reps with perfect mechanics
- Isotonic wrist, forearm, and scapular exercises.
- Theraband resisted pull-downs from the front and the scapular plane; elbow flexion with high reps and low resistance; submaximal isometrics (as dictated by pain); active scapular elevation, depression, and retraction exercises; light weight-bearing exercises.
- Upper Body Ergometer (UBE) with light to no resistance only.
- Add proprioceptive training exercises (alphabet writing, fine motor skills, work/sport-specific exercises).

Weeks 7–8

- Continue to increase active range of motion (AROM) exercises as tolerated (serratus anterior, upper and lower trapezius); add eccentrics into protected ranges.
- Okay to begin *light* stretching into external rotation.
- Okay to begin *light* glenohumeral joint mobilization.
- Okay to add light resistance internal rotation exercises from 0° to the body only.
- Increase proprioceptive training (prone on elbows, quadriped position for rhythmic stabilization).
- UBE with increasing resistance.
- Okay to begin jogging, road cycling, and standing aim resistance exercises in the pool.

Weeks 9–12

- Emphasis on regaining strength and endurance.
- Light PNF patterns (proprioceptive neuromuscular facilitation).
- AROM exercises to include internal rotation and external rotation as motion allows, lateral raises and supraspinatus isolation, rower with a high seat, decline bench press, military press in front of body.
- Running, road or mountain biking, but no activities with forceful, ballistic arm movement.

(continues)

TABLE 2.2. *Continued.*

3–6 Months

- Aggressive stretching; begin strenuous resistive exercises.
- Add light throwing exercises with attention to proper mechanics.

6 Months

- Increasing throwing program/sport-specific program with focus on return to sports as mechanics, conditioning, and strength allow.

a plan of training based on the physician's recommendations and the therapist's or trainer's own assessment. Short-term goals, such as decreasing pain, increasing general motion of the hip and pelvis through manual therapy, and improving posture through core strengthening exercises, are established. Long-term goals might include range of motion within normal limits and equal bilaterally and pain-free, sport-specific exercises.

Maintaining open lines of communication with all members of the sports medicine team improves patient outcome. Physical therapists, athletic trainers, and chiropractors usually send the physician copies of their initial evaluation as well as progress notes for periodic review. These notes are extremely useful to the physician, not only for assessing other possible contributors to the injury but also for giving input regarding the recommended treatment plan. For instance, a baseball player presents to the physician complaining of chronic shoulder pain of insidious onset with radicular symptoms and is given a diagnosis of impingement syndrome. The baseball player is referred to a physical therapist, who performs manual therapy techniques to improve glenohumeral and scapulothoracic mobility, provides postural education, and teaches stretching exercises for the shoulder capsule and intrinsic strengthening exercises for the shoulder stabilizers. During the course of care, the therapist recognizes that the athlete has underlying instability of the glenohumeral joint. The next course of action is a written progress note and follow-up discussion with the physician to determine future treatment options. At this stage the physician can intervene by reexamining the patient, confirming the diagnosis, and discussing with the athlete the options of either regular strengthening to see if this ameliorates the symptoms or surgical intervention to tighten the joint.

FINANCIAL CONCERNS

Beyond the physical and emotional concerns that injured athletes have, the source of the most significant worry is typically financial. Immediate discussions with the physician or the person in the orthopedic office who handles billing can help alleviate these sometimes needless worries and minimize their impact on the injury management process.

In the past, patients were able to focus exclusively on how they could rehabilitate their injury as quickly and effectively as possible. Today, however, in a world dominated by managed care, patients must also focus on how to overcome financial constraints to obtaining the best care. Managed care is often perceived as creating roadblocks to timely and effective treatment. How patients respond to these obstacles can affect their care and recovery. For example, some patients perceive the advice given from a generalist in sports injury care (as opposed to a specialist in sports medicine) to be "good enough" if they believe that it will save them money, whereas others are distraught over difficulty in obtaining a specialist's opinion and an immediate MRI or other advanced diagnostic study.

Understanding the patient's perception of his or her financial situation is an important first step in providing quality care that is within the means of the patient. Most important, patients should be shown what their care options are. For some patients, waiting for clearance from an insurance company for diagnostic tests or treatment is not acceptable. Typically, a timely and accurate diagnosis and the development and implementation of a treatment plan is the most immediate goal for patients and the one that generally leads to the optimal outcome.

As diagnostic and treatment options are considered, the financial burden on the patient should be taken into account. There can be many ways of treating an injury, each with its own price tag. This burden on the patient, who must balance therapeutic benefit with cost, can cause stress that can exacerbate the injury and the overall well-being of the patient. The goal is to use the most effective treatments, provide early relief, and facilitate the patient's return to sport. At the same time, the patient must choose the most effective treatment affordable. It is up to each patient to decide his or her comfort level in the treatment and financial aspects of an injury.

Patients should be queried about their sense of urgency about the injury and their financial capabilities, both within and outside the constraints of their medical coverage. Statements such as "I don't care what it costs. I want to know right now what an MRI will show" or "I am really tight on funds right now, so I would like to delay whatever I can" must be considered in determining how a physician is ultimately selected, what course of treatment is chosen, and when treatment begins. The four most important questions to have clearly answered are

- How much will the treatment cost?
- How much will insurance cover?
- How much will be out-of-pocket?
- What are the payment options?

1. *How much will the treatment cost?* Treatment costs should be detailed to include all costs that will be incurred during the entire injury management process. Costs will include physician examination and all diagnostic studies that are indicated, such as X rays, MRI, CT scans, and laboratory tests. If surgery is indicated, the injured athlete needs to know the fees for the surgeon and assistant surgeon, hospital or surgery center, anesthesiologist, supplies, and medication. Are preoperative and postoperative care from the surgeon included in the cost of surgery? If so, for how long? Rehabilitation costs will include physical therapy sessions, equipment, and home care.

2. *How much will insurance cover?* Some individuals may be fortunate enough to have insurance that allows them to choose their own physician and have treatment fully paid. More likely, however, individuals will be restricted in the amount that insurance pays, the choice of physician, or both. The best place for patients to start to get the answer to these questions is their insurance handbook—a book that very few people have taken the time to read even though they usually pay a good portion of their annual income for this coverage. The next step is a phone call to their insurance company addressing issues such as the use of "in-network" or "out-of-network" physicians, annual deductible, percentage paid by the insurance company, "usual and customary" amount for the proposed procedure, preauthorization requirements for a particular test or surgery, and the requirement for a second surgical opinion. Also, is the proposed procedure something the insurance company will pay for, or does it consider the procedure to be "investigational" or "experimental"? Careful documentation of the answers to these questions, along with the name and direct phone number of a supervisor or someone who is knowledgeable and pleasant, is useful. Finally, a skilled, conscientious, and kind billing manager who knows the system of insurance and the "ins and outs" of reimbursement is invaluable in advising patients who are overwhelmed with the financial aspects of treatment.

3. *How much will be out-of-pocket?* Deductibles and copays are typically the extent of payment required if the provider of services is in the insurance company's network. However, if the provider is not in the network, "usual and customary" amounts do not apply. This means that the patient is responsible for payment in full to the provider regardless of what the insurance company's limitations are. Also, many insurance policies put limits on the number of physical therapy visits allowed per year, and they sometimes determine that certain recommended services or supplies are not medically necessary and, therefore, do not pay for these charges. It is most important that patients completely understand the financial aspects of their treatment so that these concerns do not place undue stress on them and they can focus their time and energy on their treatment and rehabilitation.

4. *What are the payment options?* Most physicians offer a variety of payment options, including cash, check, or credit card. Some have recognized the difficulty in obtaining quality care due to financial restraints and now offer the option of a medical credit card. Patients should ask their physician if this alternative is available to them. Other relevant issues include deposit requirements and available payment plans. A creative billing manager will offer a variety of payment options and plans to suit patient needs and to ensure that patients receive the highest quality care possible in a financial arrangement that they can manage.

CHAPTER 3

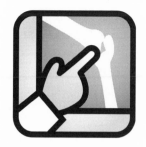

Psychological Implications of Injury

Some form of psychological distress in response to an injury is common and expected. As mentioned in Chapter 1, an injury, particularly a serious one, is highly disruptive of many aspects of an athlete's life. So, it is natural for injured athletes to experience a variety of negative emotions. It is normal for them to feel down, sad, angry, frustrated, uncertain, anxious, restless, and irritable, among other things, for several days after the injury and the initial examination. This fact should be shared with injured athletes as a means of "normalizing" what they are feeling. It is common for them to "feel bad about feeling bad," which only exacerbates their psychological distress and their negativity.

If these emotional difficulties become persistent or worsen, however, they might signal a shift from a normal, adaptive response to one that will impair the course of injury management as well as the injured athlete's general psychological and physical health. Because of this potential negative impact, members of the sports medicine team should understand the clinically significant psychological difficulties associated with injury and be alert to their manifestation. (The term *clinical reaction* or *clinical response* is used here to describe these significant psychological conditions that extend beyond normal negative psychological reactions to injury.) If an injured athlete demonstrates these clinical responses, the sports medicine team needs to know the appropriate course of action.

PREVALENCE OF PSYCHOLOGICAL DISTRESS

Psychological distress in injured athletes is a negative reaction to an injury that impairs the athlete's functioning. Low to moderate psychological distress is normal in reaction to unfamiliar, unpredictable, and uncontrollable events that occur during the injury management process. Adaptation generally results shortly after the injury as the athlete progresses to a more positive response to the injury (McDonald & Hardy, 1990). However, if adaptation does not occur, clinical reactions are likely to arise. According to the *Diagnostic and Statistical Manual of Mental Disorders* (DSM–IV), clinical reactions are seen as negative responses that significantly impair specific (i.e., related to rehabilitation) and general (i.e., other aspects of life such as school, work, and relationships) functioning (American Psychiatric Association, 1994). Clinical difficulties may be lasting and typically do not remediate without some form of professional intervention.

Considerable research has found significant prevalence of psychological distress among injured athletes. Brewer, Petitpas, Van Raalte, Sklar, and Ditmar (1995) reported a 19% prevalence rate of self-reported clinically relevant levels of psychological distress in a sample of 200 orthopedic patients, of which slightly more than half were athletes. Also, up to one third of a sample of injured football players were considered to be depressed (Brewer & Petrie, 1995).

A survey of sports medicine physicians indicated that anxiety, anger, and depression were the most frequently observed forms of psychological distress (Brewer, Van Raalte, & Linder, 1991). Two other studies found that injured athletes were significantly more depressed and anxious than noninjured athletes (Leddy, Lambert, & Ogles, 1994; Pearson & Jones, 1992). Moreover, clinical experience suggests that almost all athletes who suffer a serious injury (defined as being away from their sport for at least a month) feel some degree of psychological distress in the early stages of injury management.

PRECURSORS OF PSYCHOLOGICAL DISTRESS

Recent research indicates that there are certain precursors of psychological distress in response to injury that can act as red flags to alert the sports medicine team (Brewer, Linder, & Phelps, 1995; Brewer, Petitpas, et al., 1995; Daly, Brewer, Van Raalte, Petitpas, & Sklar, 1995). With awareness and understanding of these signs, psychological distress can be reduced with early recognition.

The appearance of psychological difficulties depends largely on the seriousness of the injury. Although athletes who sustain minor injuries, such as a second-degree sprain, may experience a transitory negative response immediately after the injury, these reactions are temporary and dissipate as soon as the athletes learn that the injury is not severe and will not keep them away from their sport for a long period. As a consequence, less attention to clinical reactions is required for athletes who have minor injuries.

Psychological distress is most common among athletes who have experienced a serious injury requiring a lengthy and potentially painful rehabilitation. For a serious injury, the pain is more severe and invasive, cessation from the athlete's sport will be longer, physical therapy will be protracted and difficult, and doubts about a full recovery will be present. The sports medicine team should closely observe athletes who have sustained a serious injury for signs of psychological distress.

How injured athletes appraise their injury is a predictor of psychological distress. Athletes who view their injury as insurmountable and hopeless are more prone to psychological distress than those who have a more positive attitude and perspective on their injury. Daly et al. (1995) asked seriously injured athletes to indicate their agreement with the statement "My injury will be difficult to deal with." Their responses were significantly related to the amount of psychological distress they experienced. Simply asking this one question can be an effective step in identifying patients who may be prone to psychological distress.

Lack of social support also appears to be a precursor to psychological distress in injured athletes. Brewer, Petitpas, et al. (1995) found that injured athletes who received insufficient social support had significantly higher levels of depression. Similarly, Brewer, Linder, and Phelps (1995) reported that injured athletes who were dissatisfied with the social support they received scored higher on a general measure of psychological distress. Pain is also related to psychological distress. Injured athletes who had significant pain experienced more psychological distress and displayed more indications of psychological difficulties (Brewer, Petitpas, et al., 1995).

Functional disability is another documented precursor to maladaptive responses to injury. Inability to engage in activities such as sports, work, and school has been significantly related to greater pain, depression, psychological distress, and behavioral manifestations of psychological difficulties (Brewer, Linder, & Phelps, 1995; Brewer, Petitpas, et al., 1995; Crossman & Jamieson, 1985). More severe injuries that lead to greater functional disability are more likely to produce psychological distress.

Research also indicates that a certain type of injured athlete is more prone to psychological distress. Athletes whose self-worth is largely defined by their sport participation are more likely to respond negatively to an injury (Brewer, 1993; Brewer, Van Raalte, & Linder, 1993). This vulnerability is accentuated when injured athletes gain little validation from other areas of their lives. Thus, the injury removes their primary, and sometimes only, source of satisfaction.

IDENTIFYING PSYCHOLOGICAL DISTRESS

Sports medicine professionals are not always aware of psychological distress in their patients (Brewer, Petitpas, et al., 1995; Crossman & Jamieson, 1985). This lack of awareness may be explained by several factors. It is easier for sports medicine professionals to observe and discuss physical states than psychological conditions. Also, sports medicine professionals receive little formal training in psychological issues arising during the injury management process, so they may not be skilled in such assessment. Finally, patients may simply not share their psychological and emotional concerns with their sports medicine team, further limiting the latter's ability to identify distress and act appropriately.

To facilitate awareness and communication of psychological and emotional aspects of patients, the sports medicine team can include observations of patients' emotional state in the patient notes. A few questions can clarify their emotional state:

- How would you describe your general attitude since your injury?
- How do you feel right now?
- How have you been emotionally since your injury?
- How do you think your recovery will affect you emotionally?

These questions can provide the sports medicine team with an overall sense on the injured athlete's general emotional state, perspective on the injury, and attitude toward what lies ahead during rehabilitation.

There are certain behaviors that indicate possible psychological distress in response to injury and rehabilitation. J. Taylor and Taylor (1997) developed the Psychological Distress Checklist (see Figure 3.1), expanding on a list of observable behaviors that suggest poor psychological reactions to injury (Gordon, Milios, & Grove, 1991). These behaviors include displaying negative emotion, avoiding acceptance of the injury and aspects of rehabilitation, resisting treatment, and not cooperating with the sports medicine team. The Psychological Distress Checklist can be useful in gauging patients' psychological conditions as they proceed through the injury management process.

The nature and severity of the emotional difficulties of injured athletes points to the need for communication between all those who are involved in the early stages of the injury management process. Transitory negative emotional responses are normal, but extended negative reactions may signal a more ongoing and potentially problematic reaction. Compartmentalized contact by the sports medicine team with little communication about the injured athletes' emotional state can result in more serious difficulties being overlooked.

IDENTIFYING SPECIFIC CLINICAL REACTIONS

Depression and anxiety are the two most commonly reported clinical reactions among injured athletes (Leddy et al., 1994; Pearson & Jones,

---

PSYCHOLOGICAL DISTRESS CHECKLIST

Directions: Place a ✓ next to each behavior that you observe on a consistent basis in a patient. The persistent presence of any of these behaviors may warrant a referral. The more items that are checked, the greater the need for a referral.

1. Not accepting injury

2. Denying seriousness or extent of injury

3. Displaying depression

4. Displaying anger

5. Displaying apprehension or anxiety

6. Failing to take responsibility for own rehabilitation

7. Not adhering to rehabilitation program

8. Missing appointments

9. Overdoing rehabilitation

10. Not cooperating with rehabilitation professional

11. Bargaining with rehabilitation professional over treatment or time out of competition

12. Frequent negative statements about injury and rehabilitation

13. Reduced effort in physical therapy

14. Poor focus and intensity in physical therapy

15. Unconfirmable reports of pain

16. Interfering behaviors outside of rehabilitation (e.g., using injured area)

17. Inappropriate emotions

18. Emotional swings

Figure 3.1. Psychological Distress Checklist. *Note.* From *Psychological Approaches to Sports Injury Rehabilitation* (p. 70), by J. Taylor and S. Taylor, 1997, Austin, TX: PRO-ED. Copyright 1997 by PRO-ED, Inc. Reprinted with permission.

1992). Both have essential implications for the quality of the injury management process as well as the normal functioning of injured athletes. It is important for the sports medicine team to have a clear understanding of the symptoms of these emotional difficulties to identify them should they be present. Moreover, they should be able to distinguish between normal emotional reactions and ones that may indicate the need for some sort of intervention.

Depression

According to the DSM–IV, the most common type of depression in response to an injury is Adjustment Disorder with Depressed Mood. The essential feature of Adjustment Disorder with Depressed Mood is "the development of emotional or behavioral symptoms in response to an identifiable stressor(s) within 3 months of the onset of the stressor(s)" (DSM–IV, p. 626). The symptoms most commonly associated with this disorder include depressed mood, tearfulness, and feelings of hopelessness. These symptoms are significant if there is "marked distress that is in excess of what would be expected from exposure to the stressor or significant impairment in social or occupational (academic) functioning" (DSM–IV, p. 626; see Table 3.1).

Other symptoms to look for in patients who are depressed include (a) changes in appetite; (b) significant weight loss or gain; (c) sleep disturbance; (d) disruption in psychomotor activity (e.g., thinking, acting, or moving more slowly or quickly); (e) decreased energy; (f) irritability; (g) feelings of worthlessness or guilt; (h) difficulty thinking, concentrating, or making decisions; or (i) thoughts of death (DSM–IV; see Table 3.1). Depression also impairs daily functioning. Depressed patients may show a loss of interest in activities and interactions that were once rewarding. They may show a decline in school or work performance. These athletes may withdraw socially from family, friends, and teammates. A significant disruption in sleep (e.g., difficulty falling asleep, waking frequently during the night, and early-morning awakening) is nearly always diagnostic of depression.

Anxiety

The most common clinical reaction to an injury is Adjustment Disorder with Anxiety (DSM–IV). The essential feature of Adjustment Disorder with Anxiety is "the development of emotional or behavioral symptoms in response to an identifiable stressor(s) within 3 months of the onset of the stressor(s)" (DSM–IV, p. 626). The symptoms associated with this anxiety disorder include nervousness, worry, and jitteriness. These symptoms are significant if there is "marked distress that is in excess of

TABLE 3.1

Factors Associated with Depressive Disorders

General Symptoms	Specific Indications
Changes in appetite or weight, sleep, and psychomotor activity	Feeling down, "bummed out," unhappy, discouraged, or hopeless
Decreased energy	Loss of motivation in rehabilitation, lack of adherence to regimen, poor effort and intensity in physical therapy
Feelings of worthlessness or guilt	Loss of confidence, negative self-talk, expressions of doubt and uncertainty, catastrophizing, feelings of worthlessness and helplessness, overall sense of inadequacy
Difficulty thinking, concentrating, or making decisions	Somatization in the form of pain and bodily discomfort
Irritability, emotional swings	Loss of interest in previously enjoyable activities and interactions
Impairment in school, work, or social relationships	Deterioration in school or work performance
Suicidal ideation; thoughts of death	Social withdrawal
Sleep disturbance	Low energy and persistent fatigue

Note. From *Psychological Approaches to Sports Injury Rehabilitation* (p. 72), by J. Taylor and S. Taylor, 1997, Austin, TX: PRO-ED. Copyright 1997 by PRO-ED, Inc. Reprinted with permission.

what would be expected from exposure to the stressor or significant impairment in social or occupational (academic) functioning" (DSM–IV, p. 626; see also Table 3.2). Specific symptoms of anxiety include restlessness, sleep disturbance, irritability, and high distractibility. Other physiological symptoms of anxiety include heart palpitations, tremors, sweating, stomach discomfort, diarrhea, muscle tension, light-headedness, and blushing (DSM–IV). Symptoms of anxiety and depression frequently coexist.

Anxiety is especially common when athletes are injured in dramatic fashion in a high-risk sport, for example, a football collision or a figure skating fall. It is typical for injured athletes to reexperience their injury in a variety of ways. Often, injured athletes with anxiety reexperience the accident persistently in the form of thoughts, dreams, images, and flashbacks, and there is an active avoidance of anything that produces memories of the event. Says Olympic skiing champion, Picabo Street, "I see it in my head over and over. I live it over and over. I'll wake up in a nightmare and I'm reliving it" ("Street Still Haunted," 1998, p. 12D).

TABLE 3.2
Factors Associated with Anxiety Disorders

Types of Anxiety	General Symptoms	Specific Indications
Adjustment Disorder with Anxiety	Nervousness	Physical symptoms of anxiety
	Worry	Negative thinking, catastrophizing of injury
	Jittery behavior	Agitation and restlessness in physical therapy
Acute Stress Disorder	Response of intense fear	Increased reports of pain
	Persistent reexperimenting of event	Preoccupation with injury
	Avoidance of related stimuli	Spontaneous replay of injury
	Symptoms of anxiety (sleep disturbance, restlessness)	Reduced ability to focus on rehabilitation
	Physical symptoms (heart palpitations, tremors, sweating, stomach discomfort, diarrhea, light-headedness, and blushing)	Muscle tension, breathing difficulties
		Emotional lability, irritability
		Displays of impatience and anger
	Impairment of normal functioning	Lack of adherence to regimen (avoidance)
Specific Phobia	Persistent, excessive fear cued by situation	Emerges as return to sport nears
	Immediate anxiety response in face of stimulus	In response to first exposure to sport postinjury
	Recognition that fear is extreme and irrational	
	Avoidance, anxious anticipation, or distress in feared situation	Same symptoms as Acute Stress Disorder
	Impairment of normal functioning	

Note. From *Psychological Approaches to Sports Injury Rehabilitation* (p. 74), by J. Taylor and S. Taylor, 1997, Austin, TX: PRO-ED. Copyright 1997 by PRO-ED, Inc. Reprinted with permission.

Anxiety affects normal daily functioning of injured athletes as well. It can lower school and work performance by interfering with concentration and clear thinking. Injured athletes experiencing anxiety often withdraw from people who remind them of the injury, for example, coaches and teammates, which acts in a counterproductive manner because it removes important sources of social support.

Other Clinical Concerns

Although depression and anxiety are the most common psychological problems that occur in response to an injury, there are other clinical reactions as well. A survey of sports medicine physicians found that exercise addiction, weight control problems, family adjustment issues, and substance abuse were observed at a moderate frequency (Brewer et al., 1991).

Exercise addiction, or the experiencing of psychological or physical withdrawal symptoms in the absence of the ability to engage in physical activity, can stem from a self-identity composed primarily of athletic identity. Absence of sufficient satisfaction and validation from other aspects of their lives can drive athletes to continue their athletic involvement to the detriment of the injury management process. Substantial weight gain or loss is another common clinical reaction, particularly for those who compete in sports with rigorous weight requirements. Gaining weight can be caused by forced inactivity associated with an injury or by overeating in reaction to depression and anxiety. Weight loss can occur in athletes who are fearful of gaining weight during rehabilitation and, as a result, reduce their calorie intake to an unhealthy level.

The clinical reaction of most concern to severely injured athletes is substance abuse. Athletes may anesthetize the emotional pain they feel by "drowning themselves" in alcohol or drugs (Tricker & Cook, 1990). Abuse of recreational drugs such as alcohol and marijuana is most common for this purpose. Abuse of pain medication may occur by accident. Reported most often with athletes suffering from serious injuries involving lengthy and painful recoveries, reliance on medication to manage injury pain may result in a psychological or physiological addiction to medication (Tricker & Cook, 1990). A telling example of abuse of pain medication is that of Brett Favre, the All-Pro quarterback for the Green Bay Packers, who developed an addiction to prescription pain medication that allowed him to play each week (King, 1996). The possible abuse of pain medication provides support for the use of nonanalgesic pain management (see Chapter 9).

REFERRAL FOR PSYCHOLOGICAL DISTRESS

When injured athletes present with symptoms of persistent psychological distress, it is essential that their difficulties be addressed in a direct and proactive manner. A timely referral to a qualified professional is critical for maintaining the quality of injury management and minimizing the harm that psychological distress inflicts on the physical and psychological health of injured athletes.

Despite this clear need, recent research has shown that, although sports medicine professionals appreciate the importance of responding to the psychological needs of injured athletes, more than 75% have never referred an injured athlete to a trained mental health professional, and only 8% had a formalized protocol for making referrals (Larson, Starkey, & Zaichkowsky, 1996). This inconsistency may be due to inadequate education in the psychological aspects of injury, insufficient time to address psychological difficulties, or the attitude that treating the physical needs of injured athletes will improve the psychological difficulties as well. It may also be that they do not adequately understand under what circumstances and at what point a referral is called for. Sports medicine professionals also may not know how to identify mental health professionals who are qualified to work with athletes through the injury management process.

In addition, many sports medicine specialists—as well as the general public—tend to see psychological distress as a temporary condition that will pass. This perspective may lead to ignoring the problem or relegating it to a low priority, which may increase distress and produce a clinical reaction. Studies indicate that untreated depression due to physical illness or injury leads to poorer medical outcomes and longer hospital stays (Franco et al., 1995). Because of the negative impact psychological difficulties can have on injury management, it is more prudent to err on the conservative side by acknowledging them and intervening.

Psychological distress manifests itself most often during the injury management process in the form of anxiety, depression, anger, pain, and treatment noncompliance. As a general rule, any psychological difficulty that persists for more than a few days and interferes with the quality of the injured athlete's treatment or daily functioning should be considered a reason for referral. More specifically, a survey of sports medicine physicians reported that family adjustment issues, substance abuse, weight control problems, depression, and exercise addiction were highly appropriate for referral, and anger and the combination of anger and anxiety were moderately appropriate (Brewer et al., 1991).

Sports medicine professionals can apply many of the same rules they use in managing physical aspects of injuries to managing psychological difficulties. For example, a patient suffers from excessive pain and swelling. Because these symptoms are common, the physician would not immediately assume a problem is present. At the same time, the presenting symptoms would not be ignored. Rather, the physician would provide appropriate treatment (e.g., analgesics and ice) and monitor the symptoms for a few days. If the problem persisted, then the physician would further examine the problem in order to find its cause.

In a similar way, during an exam, an injured athlete expresses negativity about the injury, seems depressed, and shows little interest in what the physician is saying. It is expected that injured athletes will have bad days in which they feel discouraged. The physician notes the patient's reaction and the patient's psychological symptoms are monitored for the next several days. If they do not persist, the response can be interpreted as a temporary reaction to the stresses of injury and life. However, if the maladaptive symptoms continue for more than a few days, it is a strong indication that action should be taken to address the problem.

Patient Perceptions About Referrals

The sports medicine team must go through two steps to ensure that injured athletes suffering from psychological distress are willing to seek professional help. First, the athletes must acknowledge that they are experiencing psychological distress and that it is interfering with their treatment and their general life functioning. This can be accomplished by helping them recognize and articulate what they are feeling. The sports medicine team can point out how the psychological distress is inhibiting treatment and healing. The athletes can then connect their psychological distress with difficulties they may be having in their daily lives. Once this connection is made, they will come to see that they are struggling and may be more amenable to seeking professional help.

Second, injured athletes must appreciate that a qualified mental health professional is an accepted member of the sports medicine team and a valuable resource in the injury management process. This may be difficult, because some people hold negative attitudes about seeing a psychologist or other mental health professional (Linder, Pillow, & Reno, 1989). An educational approach begun early in the injury management process can help relieve this concern. Injured athletes need to be informed about what rehabilitation psychologists do (and do not do) and how they can enhance treatment and expedite return to sport.

Early in the injury management process, the sports medicine team should make an effort to increase injured athletes' understanding of the role that psychological issues play in their recoveries, regardless of whether they are showing psychological distress or not. Like the injured area, psychological "muscles" can be damaged too and, like the sports medicine team's treatment of physical aspects of the injury, the psychologist can assist injured athletes in rehabilitating those psychological muscles.

For timely response to psychological distress, injured athletes must appreciate the value of psychological support (Brewer, Jeffers, Petitpas, & Van Raalte, 1994; Ievleva & Orlick, 1991). If they are uncertain of its value, they will be less likely to use such support, and if they do choose to try it, the intervention will most likely be less effective (Meichenbaum & Turk, 1987). Although this task may seem imposing, one study found that, following a brief educational experience, injured athletes viewed counseling as a potentially beneficial adjunct to rehabilitation and showed moderate willingness to see a psychologist if referred (Brewer et al., 1994).

Identifying a Qualified Professional for Referral

A challenge in creating an effective referral protocol is finding mental health professionals who have the qualifications and expertise to work effectively in a sports medicine setting. This concern is reflected in a survey of sports medicine physicians who questioned whether there are many psychologists capable of working with injured athletes (Brewer et al., 1991).

Mental health professionals chosen for referral should demonstrate the necessary education and training in the form of a graduate degree in clinical psychology, psychiatry, or counseling. They should also be licensed by the state in which they practice or be board certified by the appropriate medical or psychological association. Certification from relevant organizations can indicate specialized training with athletes. Potential referrals should demonstrate experience in working with common psychological difficulties that occur during injury management and preferably experience working with injured athletes. If there is no one in the area with specific experience in injury management, a psychologist or counselor who has worked in the general area of trauma, depression, or anxiety might be suitable.

There are several ways to identify qualified professionals to use as referrals. Most universities with a psychology department, athletic department, or counseling center have a professional on staff with experience in sports rehabilitation or rehabilitation in general. Also, most large hospitals have psychologists on staff who work with various departments on rehabilitation issues. There are two organizations that can be contacted to find someone qualified. The United States Olympic Committee maintains a registry of sport psychologists trained in a diverse range of areas, including injury management. For more information, contact Director of Sport Psychology, United States Olympic Training Center, 1750 E. Boulder St., Colorado Springs, CO 80908; tel: 719/578-4517; fax: 719/632-5194. The Association for the Advancement of Applied Sport Psychology (AAASP) is the largest alliance of sport psychology practitioners in the world and utilizes a certification process to establish competence criteria. For more information, contact AAASP at their Web site (www.aaasponline.org).

Developing a Referral Procedure

A clearly defined referral procedure is needed to ensure that injured athletes who experience psychological distress are able to receive timely and effective intervention so that the difficulties do not interfere with injury management (see Table 3.3). The first step in developing a referral procedure is for the sports medicine team and the psychologist to educate each other on their roles and responsibilities so that everyone understands how they can assist the others in facilitating the injury management process. Understanding each other's philosophies, approaches, attitudes, responsibilities, and specific methods will enhance the quality of the collaboration.

When the sports medicine team observes persistent psychological distress, the next step involves a telephone consultation with the referral psychologist to discuss symptoms and to obtain a professional perspective on the specific presenting problem and its likely course. If the sports

TABLE 3.3
Sample Referral Protocol

1. Identify qualified psychologist to join sports medicine team
    a. Specify and share roles and responsibilities of each sports medicine team member
    b. Have mental health professional educate sports medicine team about identification and response to relevant psychological difficulties
2. Make psychologist a member of the sports medicine team
    a. Educate injured athletes early in the rehabilitation process about importance of psychological issues in recovery
    b. Make injured athletes aware of psychologist on sports medicine team: rationale, role, and responsibilities
    c. Foster perception of "total athlete" approach to injury rehabilitation
3. Sports medicine team member observes possible psychological distress
    a. Follow course, persistence, and intensity
    b. Observe influence on rehabilitation and general life functioning
    c. Use Psychological Distress Checklist [Figure 3.1] to support observations
4. If distress is persistent
    a. Contact psychologist
    b. Describe symptoms
    c. Gain professional perspective and recommendations on presenting problem
5. Make referral
    a. Suggest value of referral to injured athlete
    b. Provide positive and constructive perspective to injured athlete
    c. Ensure communication and integrated approach between sports medicine team members (within appropriate ethical boundaries) to resolve distress

medicine team and the psychologist agree that a referral should be made, this option should be presented to the patient.

If the importance of psychological issues is emphasized from the start of injury management and mention is made that a psychologist is part of the sports medicine team and is often used to assist injured athletes in their recovery, an athlete will be more likely to view a referral as a normal and positive aspect of rehabilitation. An explanation of what the psychologist actually does can demystify the experience. Discussing the value of previous referrals with an injured athlete can also be helpful. To ensure the athelete's maximum comfort in seeing a psychologist, the role of confidentiality should also be discussed (Heil, 1993). Following are some of the psychologist's functions:

- Assists injured athletes in rehabilitating their mind along with their body

- Removes mental barriers to quality rehabilitation, such as doubt, frustration, stress, sadness, and pain

- Teaches mental skills such as goal setting, mental imagery, and relaxation training to maximize recovery

- Fosters motivation to work hard in rehabilitation

- Bolsters confidence during recovery period

- Helps maintain focus on positive and constructive aspects of rehabilitation

- Aids in overcoming emotional challenges of recovery

- Reduces loss of "competitive edge" during rehabilitation

- Assists in preparing athletes mentally for their return to sport

- Helps athletes return to or surpass their preinjury level of competitive performance

An important concern that needs to be addressed in the referral process is remuneration. No insurance companies cover psychological services within the treatment prescription, and many do not provide for psychological services at all (Brewer et al., 1991). For insurance coverage that does include psychological services, typical criteria include licensure of the mental health professional, a diagnosis that fits into a specified category, and a limit on the number of sessions. Other payment options include the medical facility's contracting with the psychologist to provide services and the injured athlete's being responsible for remuneration. All of these financial issues should be clarified in the early stages of collaboration and should be discussed with injured athletes when referral is considered.

SECTION II

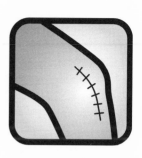

Surgery

CHAPTER 4

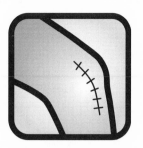

Preoperative Concerns

It has been estimated that about 1 in 10 sports injuries requires surgery. Yet, that 10% is significant because of the impact of surgery on athletes' lives. For those athletes who have not had surgery before, it is a discomforting and threatening experience that affects them on many levels. Foremost, it communicates to athletes that their injury is serious and could have long-term implications for their future athletic participation. It also tells them that they might be in for a long and painful rehabilitation. In addition, the surgery takes them into an unfamiliar realm in which they have little control and there is little predictability, thus generating more uncertainty and stress.

Particularly in a setting such as surgery, the saying "Information is power" is especially relevant. The idea of surgery to most people carries with it many fear-provoking thoughts including unconsciousness, loss of control, invasive procedures, and death. These significant worries can be allayed, if not completely alleviated, by providing injured athletes with the knowledge they need to understand the surgical process, to demystify it, and to create a sense of familiarity, predictability, and control. Taking the time to fully explain the process and answer all of a patient's questions will result in a patient who is more cooperative and less anxious, has fewer complications, experiences less pain, and has a shorter postoperative recovery time. Because of the overwhelming effects that the experience of surgery can have on injured athletes, we recommend that the information be meted out in small doses, giving patients the opportunity to process and assimilate all of it.

The goal of surgery is to foster a collaborative effort that will facilitate the injured athlete's return to health. The team builds rapport and educates the patient about what to expect before and after surgery. There are numerous questions that should be addressed to ensure that patients have a full understanding of the surgical experience. Several of the most important questions are listed in Table 4.1.

TABLE 4.1
Essential Questions Prior to Surgery

For the physician

- Does the patient understand the goals of surgery and the surgical procedure?
- Have I explained the risks in a way that is reasonable, so that if a problem arises or the outcome is not satisfactory, the patient will respond in a constructive manner?
- Have I fully empowered the patient to feel like part of the process and part of the team that will produce healing and to ultimately take responsibility for the outcome?
- Have I made it clear that the surgery is an accord between the patient, the surgeon, and the sports medicine team?

For the patient

- What are the risks of surgery?
- What anesthesia will be used and what are its side effects?
- How long will I be hospitalized?
- Will I feel pain?

For the nursing staff

- Does this patient understand the treatment process?
- Does the patient trust us to provide the best possible care?
- Are the interactions between the doctor, nurse, and office staff positive and consistent?
- Does the patient have the appropriate support to care for and assist him or her in the postoperative period?

RISKS OF SURGERY

Unfortunately, medicine is not a science of certainty. There are risks with any kind of surgery that must be understood and accepted before surgery can take place. These risks vary with the procedures. It is possible that the surgery will not improve the symptoms or, in rare cases, will make the condition worse. There may be more pain, stiffness, swelling, popping, and giving way. Nerves and vessels around the operative site may be damaged, resulting in bleeding or loss of function or sensation. There is risk of infection, blood clots, and inflammation of veins. Implants may be malpositioned or may loosen or wear out. Although rare, an allergic reaction to various substances involved in the surgery may occur. Finally, there is absolutely no guarantee of complete healing in surgery involving repair of tissues such as ligaments or cartilage. The surgeon is acutely aware of these risks and proceeds with surgical procedures in such a fashion as to minimize these risks. The patient needs to be aware of all such possibilities, however, and be prepared to work through any event.

ANESTHESIA

Anesthesia has become quite safe over the past decade as a result of improved monitoring, anesthetic techniques, and medications. However, there remain potential risks for any patient who receives anesthesia. Some are common, and others are very unlikely to occur. Reviewing the risks of the various types of anesthesia is not meant to cause alarm (only about 1 in 250,000 general anesthesia administrations results in a fatal outcome; Furlong, 2000). Rather, it is intended to educate patients about the potential problems associated with the administration of anesthesia.

The most commonly used types of anesthesia are general anesthesia, conduction anesthesia, and intravenous sedation with local anesthesia. General anesthesia, which produces unconsciousness, requires maintaining open breathing passages to ensure that oxygen and the anesthetic gases freely reach the lungs. The anesthesiologist may place one or more devices in the mouth or nose of an anesthetized patient so that the airway is unobstructed. One such airway device is an endotracheal tube, a soft, flexible, plastic tube that is inserted through the mouth and placed between the vocal cords. The tube carries oxygen and anesthetic gases to the lungs and prevents the patient's tongue from blocking the flow of these gases. Conduction anesthesia involves anesthetizing major nerves (e.g., spinal nerves or nerves to the arms or legs) with local anesthesia like novocaine. Intravenous sedation is achieved by administering sedative drugs like Valium or narcotics like morphine into the veins. This anesthetic allows the patient to be less anxious and comfortable while remaining awake. Pain or discomfort is also controlled by local anesthesia administered by the surgeon or his assistant. The decision about which type of anesthesia to use is based on a variety of factors, including type of procedure, health considerations, and the anesthesiologist's or the surgeon's preference.

Although every effort is made to minimize side effects, they are not always avoidable. The two most common are amnesia and dizziness with poor coordination, and these can occur in up to 50% of cases. Sore throat or hoarseness occurs in approximately 33%. Temporary muscle soreness occurs in approximately 8%–15% of cases. Postoperative nausea and vomiting occur in 5% of women and less than 1% of men. The following side effects occur in less than 1% of cases: pinched lips with biting of the lips or tongue, corneal abrasions, temporary or permanent nerve injuries, and damaged teeth or dental prosthetics (Atlee, 1999).

PREOPERATIVE ISSUES

As the date for surgery approaches, so does the fear. From the preoperative paperwork and medical workups, to hospital admittance, to the final surgical preparation, injured athletes know they are approaching a critical junction in the injury management process. Their fear is focused on two areas. First, the idea of surgery is anxiety provoking. Second, there is concern over whether the surgery will repair the injury. Thus, the fear is both immediate and long term. Because of the ongoing threat associated with every aspect of surgery, information is the most powerful tool physicians and the surgical staff can provide to their patients. Knowledge and understanding of everything that goes into the preoperative experience provide patients with a sense of familiarity and predictability. Having a member of the sports medicine team offer this information to the injured athlete can alleviate a number of difficulties that can arise in an already difficult situation. Also, the athlete will feel comfort in knowing that there is a member of the team who is readily accessible to assist him or her in the preoperative process.

The most intense stress over surgery usually begins the night before the procedure. Although some anticipatory stress is natural, too much is debilitating to the injured athlete psychologically, emotionally, and physically. Excessive stress may also affect the surgical outcome. If the discomfort becomes significant, patients should be given a relaxant such as Valium.

Patients usually have some questions about the preoperative routine, including (a) What exactly does the preoperative procedure entail? and (b) What do I need to do preoperatively to best prepare for the surgery? The sports medicine team—the physician, nurse practitioner, nurse, physical therapist or athletic trainer, and office or billing manager—should meet with injured athletes preoperatively, answering their questions and providing information about any pertinent matters that they fail to ask about. These interactions help patients and staff to build rapport and engender in patients trust in the sports medicine staff. This contact with the sports medicine team also lays the groundwork for continuity of care throughout the entire injury management process.

Generally, the nurse and the billing manager should meet with patients preoperatively to review the specific surgery information. During the preoperative education phase, the goal of the sports medicine team is to foster an active role on the part of the patient. The process begins by validating the patient's perception of the situation while at the same time correcting any misinformation. Treatment plans should be discussed in a collaborative fashion, and the team members should check frequently with patients to determine whether they understand what is occurring. The information that generally should be reviewed includes the following:

- The exact surgical procedure to be performed with the signing of the surgical consent

- Transportation to and from the surgery and support care during recuperation

- Instructions on the status of food and drink the night and morning before surgery—generally, nothing by mouth (NPO) after midnight the night before surgery

- Prescriptions for medications, typically to include pain and sleep medication

- Review of the icing method and protocol postoperatively, for example, a cuff or pad that is placed in the dressing at the conclusion of the procedure

- Scheduling of postoperative follow-up appointments to see the physician, nurse, and physical therapist

- Suggestions for supplies, medications, and food at home, as well as adjustments in the patient's living space to accommodate for physical limitations of the injury

- Discussion of preoperative history and physical examination

- Review of any possible machines needed for postoperative period

- Discussion of preparation of the operative area, including shaving and showering

- If the patient is nervous, finding what things might be helpful in reducing fear, such as support from family or friends, medication, music for the operating room, or talking to patients who have had a similar procedure

Close contact with patients throughout the surgical process is highly beneficial to them. We let them know that they will receive a call from the physician or nurse practitioner the evening after surgery as well as on the weekend following the surgery. Just the contact from the team and hearing that what they are experiencing is normal is very reassuring.

Patients also have considerable concern about when they can return to normal activities, such as driving, returning to work, and then returning to sports. There are no precise answers to these questions, because the time varies widely among patients. Patients are best served by the nurse's advising them of what to expect in terms of typical time (e.g., driving and returning to work: 4–10 days; reduction in swelling: 1–6 weeks; return to sport: 2–6 months depending on the procedure).

Preoperative Medication

Understandably, one of the major concerns for most patients is the management of pain. It is important for the nurse to communicate to patients that the team will make every effort to keep them as comfortable as possible. Patients commonly ask, "How much pain will I have?" A patient once wrote in a self-report to future patients, "Your recovery will not be quite the same as mine or anyone else's since we all bring different circumstances to the 'table'. . . . we all react differently to pain and discomfort, some internalizing it much more than others." What is important for patients to know is that there are many options for pain management and that there is always a member of the team available to consult with about possible medication changes.

Pain can be preemptively managed by injecting a mixture of Xylocaine or marcaine (a longer acting form of Xylocaine) into the joint before surgery to block the pain reaction before it begins. This mixture is also injected at the end of the surgery to replace any from the first dose that was washed out by the arthroscopy fluid. The patient usually receives approximately 24 hours of relative comfort from this local injection.

Another beneficial medication is Toradol, a nonnarcotic, anti-inflammatory injection that is given intramuscularly. For more extensive surgical procedures, home nursing visits up to several times a day can be arranged so that Toradol can be administered. The key to pain management is to stay on top of the pain and control it before it spirals into a more severe level that may take more medication to manage.

Preoperative Psychological Concerns

The impact of surgery on injured athletes should not be underestimated. Anticipation of surgery, following on the heels of the distress of having to face the ramifications of the injury itself, can be a threatening and potentially traumatic experience. With this in mind, particular attention from the surgeon and surgical staff should be directed toward athletes' emotional state. This awareness is very important, because considerable research indicates that a substantial portion of surgical patients experience psychological distress prior to surgery. Preoperative distress often leads to emotional difficulties following surgery. In addition, psychological distress after surgery can be harmful to the recovery process, both physically and psychologically. So, recognizing negative emotional reactions to surgery and intervening can speed recovery significantly.

The most common preoperative emotional difficulties are anxiety and depression (Leddy et al., 1994; Pearson & Jones, 1992). Moreover, these two problems have been found to be highly correlated, in that preoperative depression often leads to preoperative anxiety (Duits et al., 1999). Although there has been little research examining these issues with sport injuries that require surgery, there has been ample study of these concerns with a variety of injuries and illnesses that have analog value in considering the psychological impact of surgery on injured athletes.

Preoperative emotional reactions also have significant implications postoperatively. Studies have shown that preoperative psychological distress is highly predictive of distress postoperatively (Vingerhoets, 1998b). Patients who were depressed or anxious before surgery were more likely to be depressed or anxious following surgery (Billig, Stockton, & Cohen-Mansfield, 1996; Vingerhoets, 1998b). In addition, those patients who were both depressed and anxious prior to surgery experienced a higher incidence of depression after surgery (Timberlake et al., 1997). These emotional difficulties appear to have an ongoing negative impact on patients. For example, patients who exhibited anxiety and depression assessed their status as being much worse prior to surgery and at a 1-year follow-up than did patients who did not exhibit anxiety and depression (Perski et al., 1998).

These difficulties have been found to seriously affect many aspects of the recovery process. Depression and anxiety were reported to result in slower recoveries, greater postoperative complications, delayed wound healing, increased pain, and reduced immune functioning (Kiecolt-Glaser, Page, Marucha, MacCallum, & Glaser, 1998; Vingerhoets, 1998a).

Several studies have identified the primary contributors to psychological distress before surgery. The main cause of anxiety is concern about the success of surgery. Interestingly, detailed technical knowledge of the surgical procedure was viewed as anxiety provoking, and a substantial portion of patients did not want such an in-depth understanding of their surgery (Chaudhury, Chakraborty, Gurunadh, & Ratha, 1997). Other causes of distress include poor preparation for the surgery and inadequate education about it (Fortner, 1998).

Surprisingly, prior surgical experience increased rather than lowered anxiety among injured athletes undergoing surgery (Brewer et al., 1998). It was suggested that previous knowledge of the surgical experience increases the awareness of unpleasant aspects of the surgery and the recovery process (Langer, Janis, & Wolfer, 1975).

Recommendations for ameliorating anxiety preoperatively include having the surgeon establish a strong and supportive bond with the patient. It has been suggested that effective preoperative preparation and patient education about the surgical process and procedure also reduce anxiety and depression before surgery (Fortner, 1998). A strong doctor–patient relationship, confidence in the skills of the surgeon, and direct knowledge of a successful outcome for a similar surgery all reduced anxiety and depression (Chaudhury et al., 1997).

Although the reasons for the positive impact of the foregoing issues have not been clearly articulated, several explanations seem reasonable. As mentioned, they increase familiarity with the surgical experience, making it more predictable and giving the patient a greater sense of control over it. These perceptions, in turn, reduce the perceived threat of the procedure and increase confidence. The social support received from the physician and the sports medicine team may act as a buffer against the debilitating effects of anxiety and depression. These benefits appear to have a direct influence on patients physiologically in the form of enhanced immune activity, less pain, and facilitated healing.

A consistent recommendation that emerges from this research is the need for a systematic evaluation of patients preoperatively and identification of psychological areas that may interfere with the surgical process and recovery (Duits et al., 1999; Perski et al., 1998; Timberlake et al., 1997). This proactive approach helps identify possible emotional distress early in the injury management process, which allows for a timely and effective intervention.

It is recommended that a member of the sports medicine team complete a brief psychological evaluation of the patient prior to surgery. This may be accomplished with the psychiatric criteria and the Psychological Distress Checklist described in Chapter 3. If emotional distress is evident, its causes should be specifically identified, and solutions should be sought to relieve the difficulties before surgery.

CHAPTER 5

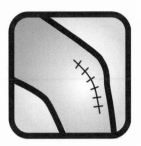

Postoperative Concerns

Upon leaving the operating room, the patient must confront the outcome of the surgical procedure. Injured athletes are especially vulnerable at this point because of the physical trauma of surgery, the anesthesia, and the pain they will begin to experience. They are also vulnerable because they are uncertain of the outcome and are experiencing a mixture of hope and apprehension as they wait for the answers to the following questions:

- What did the surgeon learn about the injury?
- How successful was the surgery?
- Were there any complications?
- What does the surgery say about the ultimate prognosis?

The answers that the surgeon gives to the injured athlete in response to these questions will "set the stage" for the athlete's immediate emotional response to the surgery as well as the athlete's initial attitude about the injury and the rehabilitation that lies ahead. A successful procedure with a positive outcome and no complications will relieve and buoy the patient. A procedure that is less successful or has complications, however, will be a serious blow to the athlete. In the latter situation, considerable effort should be made to be responsive to the athlete's immediate feelings and to quickly redirect negative feelings toward corrective options and the hope for a more positive outcome with future treatments.

To build immediate confidence in the success of the surgery, we ask the patient to exercise the limb operated on within the range permitted by the procedure as soon as the patient becomes alert. For the patient to do this successfully, we always place a large volume of local anesthetic (Xylocaine or marcaine) in the joint before leaving the operating room. The patient then can move the injured area without pain immediately. This action permits the patient to see that the injured area has been repaired. This clear physical evidence of the success of the procedure combined with positive feedback about the operation from the physician (e.g., "We were able to successfully repair it," or "There was a lot of damage but we were able to improve it") sets the stage for a positive recovery.

Once in the recovery room, patients can be given instructions on practical aspects of their postoperative experience, including when they can leave the surgical center, what to do when they arrive at home, how to diminish any pain that might arise, how much weight to bear, and when to return to the office for a follow-up appointment. This information also acts to put the procedure behind patients and lets them focus on the recovery ahead. A phone call to patients from the doctor or the nurse on the evening of surgery allays any unanticipated concerns, bolsters their confidence, and further reinforces the sports medicine team's concern for their well-being.

POSTOPERATIVE ISSUES

In some ways the postoperative experience is the most overwhelming for patients. After they leave surgery, they are faced with the unfamiliarity and physical demands of the postoperative process. Questions that often arise include the following:

- What kinds of complications might arise and what is their likelihood?
- What kinds of assistance will I need?
- How much pain will I experience and how can I manage it?
- How well will I be able to function?
- What psychological and emotional issues will I have to deal with?

Although the first two questions are important, the second two are perhaps of most concern to patients after surgery. Because most types of orthopedic surgery are highly invasive (arthroscopic surgery excepted), injured athletes can expect to experience significant pain. Moreover, this pain may be more discomforting than any they have ever faced. Even the expectation of this pain can cause stress and tension that may exacerbate the pain. Providing patients with pharmacological and nonpharmacological means of pain management can have both physical and psychological benefits.

Additionally, injured athletes will be temporarily incapacitated after surgery and in the early stages of recovery. The degree of disability will depend on the area of the injury and its severity. For example, knee surgery will severely limit mobility, whereas shoulder surgery may only inhibit use of one arm. This incapacity can be especially problematic for athletes because they are often accustomed to high levels of ability rather than inability. Thus, their temporary limitations in functioning will have both a physical impact and a psychological and emotional effect on them.

A second key factor in optimizing a patient's postoperative experience is the education and coordination of members of the sports medicine team who will be involved in the patient's care. A carefully orchestrated postoperative procedure is one in which every member of the team works in unison with one another. Communication among all caregivers—surgeons, nurses, physician assistants, and physical therapists—is critical to keep the process as efficient as possible. Keeping the tone of the environment professional, coordinated, and caring, with some degree of levity, makes the experience more effective and enjoyable for the patient.

Written protocols and morning briefings improve consistency in the information that is being given to the patients. Few things make a patient more anxious postoperatively than not being certain of precautions and restrictions. Patients need to be sure of what they should and should not be doing, how often or how long they should continue with some of the instructions, or when they can engage in relevant postoperative activities such as weight-bearing, showering, driving, and using stairs. Because of the amount of information the patient needs to digest, having written handouts for all reviewed information will aid in compliance. This consistent communication begins preoperatively, continues in the recovery room, and is maintained through the later stages of a patient's recovery.

RECOVERY ROOM

The recovery room is a large area specifically designed to treat a number of different postoperative patients at the same time, under the assumption that their individual needs will be similar. It is supervised by nurses whose primary job is to allow for patients to wake from surgery as comfortably as possible. The nurses tend to the patients' needs while they are recuperating, and they ensure that the patient is stable and strong enough to leave the surgical facility.

For patients who have surgery under general anesthesia, once they wake from their surgery, their first thought usually occurs in the recovery room. Patients who have undergone surgery under general anesthesia awaken with various levels of coherence. Some patients wake up lucid, fully aware of what they have just been through. Others come out of anesthesia groggy and require time to orient themselves to their surroundings and their surgical experience.

Once patients awake, they have some kind of "proof" that they underwent a procedure—a bulky dressing on their surgical repair site, perhaps a brace or a sling, a cold therapy unit, drains, or even a CPM (continuous passive motion) machine. This is their first recognition of some level of impairment. Some patients will remember parts of the procedure and will be cognizant of what has occurred. Mental preparedness and the bedside manner of the recovery room team can significantly aid in the physical and psychological comfort of the patient.

Patients who have surgery under a local anesthetic with intravenous sedation or epidural anesthetic are usually coherent postoperatively. The local anesthetic acts simply to alleviate localized pain. Most discomfort immediately after surgery is usually due to the positioning of the extremity during surgery or soreness from manipulation of the joint. Sometimes the use of a leg holder, a pneumatic tourniquet, or an assistant's grip to stabilize a limb can cause postoperative soft tissue soreness and bruising.

How patients respond on awakening from surgery often dictates their initial attitude toward their recovery. Now is the time when a positive mental outlook, a future focus, and motivation toward recovery are essential. It is all too easy for patients at this stage to acquiesce to self-pity. Most patients are in an impressionable state postoperatively and can be easily influenced—either positively or negatively. Patients will look to the sports medicine team to determine how they should respond immediately following surgery. This reaction often sets the tone for their subsequent rehabilitation and recovery. The postoperative time is an excellent opportunity for the sports medicine team to instill the positive attitude that is so essential to recovery.

Of particular importance is the visit from the surgeon while the patient is in the recovery room. The postoperative report from the surgeon can have a lasting impression. For many patients, despite any feedback about the surgery that they may receive from the nurses and the staff, they will not feel relief and confidence in the surgical outcome until they hear from the surgeon that it was a success. Although it is not uncommon for patients who underwent general anesthesia not to recall the visit, they do retain the overall positive feeling of the meeting. Additionally, family and friends who accompanied the patient to the surgery get a chance to hear from the physician and further instill the positive orientation in the patient.

Also relayed to patients in the recovery room is the bulk of the information about how to care for their surgical site for the first few days until they are seen by the surgeon again. Information on the dressing and surgical bandages, icing, compression and elevation, and things to watch for (e.g., high fever, excessive sweats, increased drainage) are all reviewed with the patients and their family or friends at this time.

ANTI-INFLAMMATORY AND PAIN MEDICATION

Physicians have a number of medications at their disposal that play a central role in the initial care of most acute and chronic injuries. The purpose of these medications is to facilitate healing through controlling pain and reducing inflammation. Medications commonly used include (a) nonsteroidal anti-inflammatory drugs, or NSAIDs (e.g., aspirin, ibuprofen, naproxen, diclofenac, ketoprofen, etodolac, nabumetone, rofecoxib, and celecoxib), (b) nonnarcotic analgesics (e.g., acetaminophen), and (c) corticosteroids (e.g., methylprednisone), which are typically injected into joint spaces.

Physical trauma is one force that induces the body to produce an inflammatory response. Ultimately, the response acts to remove cellular debris and prepare the area for tissue repair. This is initiated by the release of chemical mediators that trigger vascular and cellular changes. Unfortunately, these changes contribute to symptoms such as swelling, redness, pain, and loss of motion and function. When anti-inflammatory medications are consumed early after surgery, they may limit this inflammatory response and in turn limit such symptoms. However, these drugs may also impair or delay the healing response.

NSAIDs affect some of the chemical mediators that trigger vascular and cellular changes. Prostaglandins and leukotrienes are derived from arachidonic acid in the body during an inflammatory response and potentially influence each step of the inflammatory process. NSAIDs primarily affect the enzymes necessary for the production of prostaglandins, COX I and COX II enzymes. These drugs inhibit prostaglandin synthesis, reducing the inflammatory response. Their analgesic effect is an added benefit to their use.

Choosing the appropriate medication is not always easy. These medications vary in cost, side effects, effectiveness, and dosing schedules. Aspirin is considered the prototype for NSAIDs; however, some patients are unable to tolerate the gastrointestinal side effects. Alternative compounds generally produce less gastrointestinal side effects, but these drugs also have similar toxicities and may interact with other medications that the patient may be taking.

Nonnarcotic analgesics, such as acetaminophen, inhibit prostaglandin synthesis in the central nervous system—accounting for their ability to reduce pain and fever. However, their ability to effect prostaglandin synthesis in the peripheral tissues is minimal. Therefore, acetaminophen is effective as an analgesic, and because it has fewer side effects, it is better tolerated by most patients.

Systemic corticosteroids inhibit both prostaglandin and leukotriene synthesis, unlike NSAIDs, which are able to inhibit only prostaglandins. Experimentally, corticosteroids can inhibit all phases of inflammation. Unfortunately, the threat of adverse side effects of systemic use restricts their use in the injured patient. However, when corticosteroids, like methylprednisolone, are injected locally into the joint spaces, they can interrupt the inflammatory process in acutely irritated tissues or joints. Their effect may give permanent or merely temporary relief. Intraarticular injections still have risks, including weakening of the tissue, further acceleration of an underlying disease process, or infection.

The foregoing medications treat symptoms. Researchers are trying to develop agents that can prevent and repair damaged tissue. A potentially promising agent is glucosamine sulfate. Glucosamine is a subcomponent of cartilage, synovial fluid, intervertebral disks, lung tissue, vessel walls, and intestinal mucosa. It is reported to inhibit the breakdown of proteoglycans, the ground substance of articular cartilage. It has been shown to have chondroprotective and antiarthritic effects as well as a mild anti-inflammatory effect. Clinically, glucosamine has decreased patients' pain, joint tenderness, and swelling. In fact, some studies have shown glucosamine to be as effective or more so than some anti-inflammatories; however, it tends to have a slower rate of pain reduction. Glucosamine also is often better tolerated than anti-inflammatories.

POSTOPERATIVE SUPPLIES AND TREATMENTS

Dressings

After an operation, the patient's surgical site is closed and covered with porous, transparent strips that keep the surgical incision(s) closed. The strips are covered with a sterile combine dressing that soaks up bleeding from the surgical site and also acts as a barrier. A bulky dressing serves several functions. It holds all of the underlying dressings, provides extra compression at the surgical site, aids in resorption of increased draining, and holds any drains or a cold-compression bladder in place. This secondary dressing also has an added benefit in that the patient does not have to actually see the appearance of the area and perhaps develop a negative mental image.

Proper care of the postoperative dressing is paramount in optimizing wound healing, reducing soft tissue fibrosis at the surgical site, and preventing infection. The dressing can be loosened and tightened periodically as needed because of a poor fit or swelling by merely unwrapping the covering and reapplying. Care should be taken to reduce pulling of the healing tissue by a loose dressing. Due to the introduction of anesthetic medications into the area, significant pulling on any surgical incisions may not be accompanied by pain. The fit of the dressing should be carefully monitored, especially if the patient is weight-bearing or is ambulatory.

Compression and Elevation

The benefits of adequate compression and elevation in treating wounds and soft tissue injury are well documented (Arnheim, 1989; Prentice, 1986, 1999; Schurman, Goodman, & Smith, 1990; Wilk, 1999). It has been suggested that compression in and of itself may be superior to all other modalities for controlling hemorrhage, edema, and hematoma formation (Arnheim, 1986b, 1989). Although this inflammatory phase is essential to healing, maintaining stasis of the release of these exudates (i.e., plasma proteins) into the intercellular spaces is critical. Prompt resolution of this initial phase is important. If this stage is not allowed to be completed promptly, then further tissue cell necrosis may occur due to remaining devitalized tissue in the area and lack of repairs to the site by the leukocytes and prostaglandins (American Academy of Orthopaedic Surgeons, 1991; Prentice, 1986; Schurman et al., 1990). A chronic inflammatory response may occur, resulting in continued pain and swelling at the surgical site and increased atrophy of the surrounding musculature. Most of the postoperative strategies are designed to help the surgical repair site to progress rapidly through this initial inflammatory phase to normal healing.

Drains

The use of drains in the surgical site is a controversial issue. The rationale for their use is to control the initial inflammatory response and to remove any excessive bleeding, irrigation fluids, and saline from the surgery itself. In general, the use of drains is declining as data suggest that healing is not improved by their use; they can also be painful. The drain is usually wrapped in the dressing and removed at the next postoperative visit (usually the next day if a drain is used). Removal is performed by first educating the patient as to what is to happen, then extracting the tube with one quick pull in the direction it was inserted. It has often been described as feeling like a snake being pulled out of the leg. Some patients recollect this moment as one of the more uncomfortable feelings of the postoperative process.

After surgery, it is important to keep the surgical site as pristine and free from outside germs as possible. We have found that as long as the area has been suitably drained of fluid intraoperatively, complete sterile measures have been followed, and all tissue has been sufficiently closed with sutures and properly wrapped with a compressive dressing, then the risk for infection or postoperative bleeding is minimized.

Cold Therapy

Numerous studies have been published about the benefits of cold therapy early in the postoperative process (American Academy of Orthopaedic Surgeons, 1991; Arnheim, 1986b; Ho, Coel, Kagawa, & Richardson, 1994, 1995), although there still continues to be some disagreement as to how much, how often, and for how long it should be used. The use of cold therapy is effective in reducing edema, draining, and hemorrhaging. One study compared the effects of blood flow to the knee after topical application of ice for 20 minutes and found that metabolism of cells in tissues around the knee decreased by 19.3% and soft tissue blood flow by 25.8% (Ho et al., 1994). This is significant when discussing treatment options and reduction of fluid seepage into the surrounding tissue. It also has a secondary effect on the reduction of postoperative use of narcotics and pain medications.

For edema control to be most effective, cold therapy treatments must be instituted within 30 to 60 minutes after surgery. If conventional ice bags are used, 30-minute sessions every 1–2 hours are most effective for the first 2–4 days. Care should also be taken to avoid saturation of the dressings from condensation—using an unfolded garbage bag as a barrier works well. If a cold therapy device is utilized, it can be used fairly continuously for the first 1–2 days, but the patient should be warned not to allow for too much compression. After that time, use the "3–5 Rule": ice the area 3–5 times a day, for 30–50 minutes at a time, for 3–5 days. It is important to allow about 2 hours between icing sessions for optimal tissue homeostasis.

Braces, Splints, and Casts

The patient may need some kind of support to stabilize the surgical site or restrict the amount of movement. In severe cases of trauma, the patient may require an external fixator, a device pinned to a fracture site from the outside to allow for incremental changes in the amount of tension on the site.

In other cases, a brace, splint cast, or sling may be warranted to restrict motion and to protect the surgical site. For example, in a repair of the shoulder rotator cuff or labrum, if excessive motion takes place too early in the healing phase, the sutures or anchors may be pulled out. Excessive accessory motion can cause secondary damage by continuously pulling on the surgical site, causing the area to heal too lax. For this reason, surgeons prescribe anything from sling use postoperatively to use of an immobilizer that holds the arm to the side of the body. An abduction pillow may be used to immobilize the shoulder and allow for healing of the tissue in the shortened state. The choice is based on the extent of the repair, how the repair was carried out, and physician preference.

Another case that might warrant a brace is knee surgery. If a standard arthroscopic procedure was carried out without suture repair of tissue or reconstructive elements, then there is no need to immobilize the area. However, in more complex cases of ligament reconstruction or cartilage repair, most often a knee brace is used to restrict any range of motion, to remind the patient not to overuse the area, or to protect the knee from unexpected trauma. Ultimately, the decision whether to use braces or other types of support is based on extant research and the surgeon's experience and preference.

Continuous Passive Motion Machines and Foot Pumps

A continuous passive motion (CPM) machine is a device that supports a limb and moves it passively through a preset range of motion to optimize healing of an injured area. There are units designed for the knee, shoulder, ankle, wrist, and even the hallux. Research is inconclusive as to whether CPM use following anterior cruciate ligament (ACL) reconstruction surgery is beneficial, although CPM has been shown to abet healing in articular cartilage resurfacing techniques such as microfracture and in articular cartilage transplantation. Several factors may influence a surgeon's decision to use CPM: the amount of research indicating its use, availability of a CPM machine, the surgeon's professional experience, and the surgical procedure performed.

A foot pump is another machine sometimes used after surgery. Although its use is relatively rare in the sports medicine environment, it does have some indications in severe trauma cases, which typically cause more extensive swelling. Foot pumps are designed to enhance blood flow in the legs. Utilizing a compressive foot pad, the pump repetitively squeezes and releases, compressing the dorsal pedal artery and the lymphatic system in moving swelling and bleeding out of the lower leg. Foot pumps are an effective defense against the development of deep-vein thrombophlebitis.

Crutches and Assistive Walking Devices

In surgical cases involving the lower extremity, the use of crutches following surgery is usually indicated. Using an assistive walking device early in the postoperative stage helps protect the surgical repair site, improves mobility, and reduces stress on other areas of the body. When a surgeon instructs a patient on the use of crutches, it is imperative that the surgeon give verbal—and preferably written—instructions on weight-bearing status. Crutches should be properly fitted to avoid placing abnormal stresses on the body. It is best to meet with patients before surgery whenever possible to properly fit them for any assistive walking devices and educate them on their use.

SUPPORT AND ASSISTANCE

Support from significant others such as family and friends is crucial in the recovery process and usually starts when they visit the patient in the recovery room. It is difficult to know how much a patient will want to do or be able to do for himself or herself following surgery, so it is best to arrange for constant care or company for at least the first few days following the procedure.

Support is physical, practical, and emotional: giving massages, filling ice trays, making a meal, consoling, motivating, and so forth. It is important for the support person to always remain calm and comforting because the patient may "feed" off the support person's nervousness or become annoyed with it. Personal support coupled with the support of the sports medicine team help the patient to realize that he or she is not alone in the process and that there is always some type of help available. The issue of support is discussed in more detail in Chapter 10.

GETTING HOME

When patients are released from the surgical facility, they are typically discharged in a wheelchair. In most cases, patients have been instructed to arrange for someone to drive them home. Presurgery planning includes arranging the household to make the patient as comfortable as possible. If the patient is recovering from shoulder or upper-extremity surgery, tasks such as opening bottles, doing dishes, and showering can be difficult. In lower-extremity surgery—especially if there are weight-bearing restrictions—making meals, pouring a drink and carrying it to a table, and going to the bathroom can be challenging.

Making sure that the home is adequately prepared for the worst-case scenario is always best. That is, plan on the patient's being very debilitated and in a lot of pain and having very limited mobility. Following are some of the more basic issues to consider when preparing the home for a surgical patient:

- Extra pillows to support upper back and arm or leg

- Extra gauze and bandages for reinforcement

- Try to fill any prescriptions beforehand

- Pitcher of water next to the bed or couch

- Ice for cryotherapy machines or ice bags

- Grocery shopping for a week

- Prepared meals in refrigerator and freezer for easy reheat

- Move bedroom to main floor to avoid stair use

- Reading or writing material, laptop, or television or radio easily accessible

- If pets, make sure that a friend can come to the house to help tend to their needs

Any medical devices prescribed for home use will also need to be readied for postoperative care. CPM machines, foot pumps, and cryotherapy units should be free from any loose wires, bad connections, or old extension cords and set up in a convenient location where the patient will be recuperating. Making sure that the residence has adequate voltage is also a consideration in some cases.

If a machine malfunctions, the manufacturer is responsible for its upkeep. A good precaution is to provide the patient with relevant phone numbers so that problems can be resolved quickly and not interfere with recovery.

In most cases, the patient will have been instructed on some form of exercises or general care that should be adhered to in the first few days. In some cases, it will be nothing more than icing and elevation. In other cases, a more extensive home program of stretching and exercises will be reviewed. Figures 5.1 and 5.2 give sample programs for general care of the shoulder and knee, respectively, for the first few days after arthroscopic surgery. These are general protocols that can be modified based on specific diagnosis.

Sling use

>   As needed or comfortable for the first 2–3 weeks.

Icing

>   Use the shoulder icing pad or cuff regularly throughout the day for the first 3–5 days.

Posture

>   Practice good postural habits regularly (e.g., sitting/standing up straight; avoid military posture). This helps aid in healing as well as reduces stress on the repair.

>   Five times a day, sit up straight and squeeze shoulder blades together. Hold 5 seconds and repeat 10 times.

>   Probably most comfortable to sleep semireclined for the first 1–2 weeks.

Putty grips

>   Squeeze putty or soft ball regularly throughout the day.

Elbow flexion/extension

>   Three to five times a day take arm out of sling and flex and extend elbow 10–20 times in front of body. This is to prevent the elbow from becoming stiff.

Pendulums

>   Standing bent over with nonoperative hand supported on a chair or table, relax operative arm and let it dangle. Rotate through the body to swing arm around in circles clockwise, counterclockwise, forward/back, and side-to-side two to three minutes 5 times a day.

Range of motion

>   Lying on back, grasp left wrist with right hand and lift up overhead until tight. Perform 10 repetitions 5 times a day.

Aerobic exercise

>   Okay to use the stationary bike and stair machine (without weight on arms).

>   Nonsurgical arm and leg weight training also okay, making sure not to overstress the surgical shoulder.

Figure 5.1. Shoulder arthroscopic surgery initial postoperative program, Days 1–5.

Icing and elevation

Ice and elevate regularly throughout the day and night. Elevation needs to be as high above the level of the heart as is practical.

If using a cryotherapy unit, use as much as comfortable for the first day, then 30- to 60-minute sessions 3–5 times a day. Make sure to use a pillowcase between the skin and ice cuff. If using ice bags, do 20- to 30-minute sessions every 2 hours using a garbage bag as a barrier to avoid condensation.

Weight bearing

If partial weight bearing is indicated, use the crutches to assist walking until physician clearance for full weight bearing has been given. Touch down the crutches when the surgical leg is on the ground, and walk through with a particular emphasis on a stable midstance and smooth roll-through.

If weight bearing is not indicated, then crutches should be used to avoid placing any weight on the surgical side. Once the legs swing through, then land on the heel of the nonsurgical side.

Stretching (if no range-of-motion restrictions)

Every hour, go through a routine of extension and light flexion stretching. Each stretch should be held 30 seconds and repeated 5–10 times.

Sitting on the floor with your heel on a pillow, both hands on your thighs, and your leg relaxed, slowly push straight down on your thigh to stretch your leg out into extension.

Grasp the back of your thigh and bring your leg toward you to flex the knee into bend. Go until it just gets tight—do not overbend.

Exercises (if indicated)

- *Quad sets*

  Either sitting on floor with leg out straight in front or sitting on the edge of a chair with the heel on the floor, tighten thigh muscle, focusing on the inner thigh. Hold 5 seconds and repeat 10 times.

- *Leg raises*

  Start with sets of 10 repetitions and work up to 4 sets of 25 repetitions. This exercise can be done all at once or broken up throughout the day. Make sure to actively lift and lower the leg and not let momentum do the work.

  Lying back on elbows with nonsurgical knee bent, lift surgical leg up to the level of the opposite knee.

  Lying on nonsurgical side with bottom leg bent, actively lift surgical leg to the side, keeping foot parallel to the ground.

(continues)

Figure 5.2. Knee arthroscopic surgery initial postoperative program, Days 1–5.

- *Leg raises (continued)*

  Lying on stomach, lift leg up behind you without arching back.

  Lying on surgical side, step opposite leg over so that the foot is flat on the ground in front, lift surgical leg up and inward, keeping it parallel to the ground.

Figure 5.2. *Continued.*

POSTOPERATIVE COMPLICATIONS

Orthopedic surgery is designed to improve the overall function of an injured area and return it to its original state. In deciding whether to operate, there are a few things to consider. One of the very bases of medicine is, first, do no harm. There is always a risk that surgery will aggravate the injury. The patient should be prepared for surgery both physically and mentally. Physically, has the injured area had the opportunity to heal from the initial trauma? Additionally, any hot, swollen, or irritated limb—unless it is the trauma itself causing it—should be treated conservatively until it is less symptomatic. Mentally, has the patient been able to recover from the initial shock of the injury? The patient must have a positive orientation to constructively handle the trauma, pain, and rehabilitation that go with surgery.

Pain

Because perceptions of pain are highly subjective, it is difficult to tell patients the degree of pain they may experience after surgery. It can be reasonably expected that there will be some level of discomfort to the area. The patient's previous experience with injuries and pain can act as a guide to his or her level of pain tolerance. Certainly, the nature of the procedure performed has a significant impact on the level of discomfort postoperatively. Clinical experience with the procedure being performed and the feedback from other patients who underwent the same procedure can serve as a guide to the degree of pain to expect. Describing some of the sensations and symptoms the patient may feel after surgery can dramatically reduce fears and apprehension, and often reduces perceived levels of pain.

Pain has an essential role in the injury rehabilitation process. It has both a positive and negative impact on the healing process and should be viewed as a tool in determining progress. With excessive pain comes increased tension of the area, increased worry that things are not progressing well, reduced healing to the area, development of compensatory patterns in day-to-day activities, and a subsequent decrease in motivation to progress with the rehabilitation. Understanding the difference between pain and tightness to the area is an important tool in dealing with postoperative pain. The ability to differentiate between general pain and discrete, localized tissue injury is helpful in guiding the intensity of activities after an operation.

Hyper- or hyposensitivity to pain can both be problematic. Hypersensitivity is usually associated with low pain tolerance. It has been observed that patients who are anxious, dependent, and immature have less tolerance for pain than those who are relaxed and in control (Arnheim, 1989). This population, in particular, benefits from education and recognition of pain areas. The more they can be informed of the kinds of pain they will feel and how they can reduce the pain, the better they will be at tolerating the pain. General care of patients with hypersensitivity to pain should consist of more concrete scheduling of treatment approaches. Giving a written schedule of *exactly* when to ice, elevate, take the pain medication, exercise, and even perform tasks of daily living reduces the incidence of excessive pain due to poor monitoring and also enhances patients' sense of control over their pain.

Making things even more clinically challenging are incidences in which there is some doubt as to whether there is true pathology in the area where the patient senses the most amount of pain. In these incidences, meticulous care should be taken to obtain a thorough history, perform a comprehensive clinical examination, and order adequate tests to confirm the diagnosis. Thorough documentation is of the utmost importance as well. The patient's chart must reflect a logical treatment algorithm along with proper execution of all treatment approaches.

Hyposensitivity to pain presents another clinically challenging situation in that the patient could be doing significant damage to the surgical site without being aware of it. This too provides the opportunity for the sports medicine team to significantly reduce postoperative complications by increasing patient understanding and compliance. The more patients understand what will be happening surgically and what could be done to damage the injured area postoperatively, the more likely they will be to adhere to the postoperative plan. This can be best accomplished by making patients active participants in their rehabilitation. Patients must recognize that further injury can occur at the acute level, for example, with a fall onto the surgical site or with excessive accessory motion to a repaired area. Hyposensitive patients also benefit from careful supervision of a controlled postoperative treatment protocol.

Infection

Even though surgery is performed under strict sterile conditions, there is always a risk of infection. During surgery, any incisions are closed with absorbable sutures for the deeper layers of tissue and with nonabsorbable sutures for the skin. The area is covered with a sterile dressing and, usually within the first few hours, reaches some level of stasis. However, anything from inadequate sterilizing techniques during surgery, nonsterile procedures in the postoperative phase, individual metabolism, or nutritional considerations can cause some level of local irritation or infection.

If infection is suspected, a careful examination should be undertaken to determine its presence and cause. If there is drainage, a wound culture should be taken. The area should be rebandaged, with special care taken to ensure the sterility of the cleansing and proper application of topical antibiotics. It is not uncommon for patients to develop a local rash or raised tissue as a result of the iodine used to prep the area for surgery. This does not denote an infection, but rather merely a topical reaction.

When a member of the sports medicine team evaluates the patient for a possible infection, his or her demeanor and response can often set the stage for how the patient will respond. It is important that the person know how to evaluate with a poker face, without making facial expressions that might cause the patient undue concern and anxiety. Even if there is cause for alarm, the patient should merely be informed of the potential gravity of the situation and the necessary treatment and not left thinking that there is cause for alarm. The team member conducting the evaluation should exercise discretion when informing the patient of the results of the evaluation, for example, using words such as *irritation* as opposed to *infection*. There is a negative connotation associated with any statement indicating infection, and the patient might magnify the problem. Therefore, it is best that the patient be carefully educated as to how to treat the wound and guided toward a successful outcome, with any unnecessary concern being avoided.

Falls

Another major concern following surgery is the risk of a fall onto the surgical site. For lower extremity injuries, careful instruction should be given on the use of assistive walking devices such as crutches or a cane. For other injuries, patients should be impressed with the need to protect the repaired area from any form of trauma. It is preferable to inform patients of this before surgery so that they have the opportunity to practice without the influence of pain or compromised balance. In particular, going up and down stairs, navigating slick surfaces, and making technique-oriented adjustments (e.g., with crutches, avoiding too much weight through the hands, making sure auxillary pads are sufficiently under shirt and not caught on the sleeve, maintaining good posture) should be mastered before releasing patients on their own.

Educating patients about when they are susceptible to falls also reduces the risk of getting caught off guard. For instance, it is not uncommon for postoperative patients to get light-headed and even pass out if they get up too quickly when they have been sitting or lying down. Educating patients to give themselves adequate time to get up and let their body adjust can further reduce the likelihood of this occurrence. Sudden surface changes (e.g., from carpeted to tile floor), being seated at a desk, and weather changes (e.g., rain, ice, or snow) are other examples of situations when patients are more susceptible to falling.

If a fall does occur, patients often do their best to protect the surgical site from trauma. It is not uncommon to hear of willful falls onto a hip or a roll onto the opposite side to avoid direct impact on an area. Knowing in advance what positions can damage the surgical site also helps avoid impact at the site. For example, if someone who has undergone shoulder stabilization surgery were to fall, it would be better for the person to tuck in the arm and roll than to use the arm to break the fall, because the latter would involve too much rotation or shear force at the repair site.

Even more challenging is evaluating a surgical site after a fall. In most incidences, the area is already swollen and tender, and often it cannot be thoroughly evaluated with special tests, because they might put too much stress on the repaired tissue. This is when optimal clinical decision making is critical. Taking as accurate a history as possible about the fall and the position the patient landed in is helpful. Was there a twist of the limb on the way down? Was there direct impact at the site? Were there any noises, such as a pop, snap, or crack? Was there an immediate increase in the amount of swelling? Current level of pain can also provide valuable clues as to the degree of trauma. Considerable pain lasting for a few minutes and then subsiding with only minor soreness suggests that no serious damage occurred. However, if pain persists following a fall, there is gross effusion, or there is stinging pain that comes and goes—especially at rest—then more significant damage should be suspected.

Treatment should consist of first determining whether there is damage to the surgical site. X rays may be needed to determine position of fixation devices, and possibly even an MRI if it is ascertained that the results will not be skewed by any hardware or excessive swelling. Palpation and special testing can often reveal underlying pathology, but if the patient is exceptionally tender or guarding, reevaluation in a few days may be necessary. Any incisions should be carefully examined for discharge from the site or disruption of the incisions or sutures. Basic RICE (rest, ice, compression/crutches, elevation) principles for edema and pain control, and modification of postoperative protocol, should be carried out to accommodate for any trauma caused by the fall. The patient should also be carefully educated as to signs of anything more serious over the following 24–48 hours.

Deep-Vein Thrombosis

There is risk of deep-vein blood clots following extremity surgery. Although more common in more extensive open surgeries, such as total knee or total hip replacement surgery, there is a danger of developing a vessel clot in any surgical case. The literature varies on the incidence of deep-vein thrombosis in orthopedic surgery except in the total joint population, but it has shown anywhere from a 2% risk for low-risk patients undergoing minor procedures to between 50% and 70% for high-risk patients undergoing major surgery (Huo & Harrison, 2000). Several factors appear to play a role in the susceptibility of a patient to deep-vein thrombosis. Previous history of blood clots, major surgery (longer than 1 hour and with open arthrotomy or significant drilling or fracture sites), obesity, use of oral contraceptives, and metabolic factors such as deficiencies in antithrombin or proteins C or S can increase a patient's risk of developing deep-vein thrombosis (Huo & Harrison, 2000).

Prevention and early intervention are essential when dealing with deep-vein thrombosis. Practicing general RICE principles is the first defense in preventing excessive inflammation of the surgical area. Compressive stockings are often used, although much more frequently with lower extremity surgery than upper extremity. They are an effective means for providing circumferential compression to the area. Also known as TED hoses, they slide up from the foot to either the calf or thigh for lower extremity surgery, or from the hand up the arm to the shoulder in upper extremity surgery. For a lower extremity injury, patients should combine elevation with regular intervals of foot pumps in which the patient dorsiflexes and plantarflexes the foot up and down 50–100 times every waking hour. Exercising the entire limb when possible also helps control edema by mobilizing the fluid out of the tissues. Figure 5.3 describes a series of movements aimed at more efficiently moving tissue fluids.

---

1. *Perform 10 repetitions of each exercise every waking hour.*
2. *Any areas of restricted movement by surgery should be avoided, but the rest of the sequence should be continued.*

Lower Extremity Surgery
    Curl and spread toes
    Pump foot up and down
    Bend and extend knee
    Tighten thigh (leg does not need to be straight)
    Tighten gluteal muscle
    Tighten abdominal muscles by pulling in on stomach muscles

Upper Extremity Surgery
    Curl and extend fingers
    Bend and extend wrist
    Make a tight fist
    Bend and extend the elbow
    Tighten upper arm
    Move arm up and down
    Tighten pectoral (chest) muscles

Figure 5.3. Optimal edema control.

Arthrofibrosis

Arthrofibrosis is best defined as "a condition of restricted motion characterized by dense proliferative scar formation, in which intra-articular and extra-articular adhesions can progressively spread to limit joint motion" (Lindenfeld, Wojtys, & Husain, 1999, p. 1778). Usually precipitated by injury or surgery, this condition can cause significant loss of motion and subsequent decreased function.

Patients with arthrofibrosis are often much slower in gaining their range of motion following surgery and become accomplished "compensators" when using the injured limb. Pain is usually excessive, and patients often begin to use the limb in a fixed or locked pattern of movement. Patients typically present with a joint that is swollen, stiff, and often disproportionately painful or guarded with attempted range of motion. The symptoms may come on very quickly, with the patient sometimes losing up to 60%–70% of range of motion within a few weeks following surgery despite rehabilitation.

Treatment is fairly straightforward, with rehabilitation targeting decreasing pain, improving range of motion, and increasing functional capacity. Manual therapy techniques consisting of soft tissue mobilization of the surrounding structures along with joint mobilization are effective at restoring normal joint kinematics, increasing range of motion, and reducing pain. Ice, elevation, and modified activity are also effective in reducing symptoms. Oral anti-inflammatory medications may be helpful if there is an acute inflammatory response. Aspirations of any chronic effusions are also beneficial. Making sure the patient is on a comprehensive home treatment program is the other key element to promote improved mobility and function with such a condition.

Reflex Sympathetic Dystrophy

Trauma to the sympathetic nervous system can present in different ways. Most often insidious in development, it can have relatively mild symptoms with only transitory indications or more extensive regional pain dysfunction. Reflex sympathetic dystrophy is a "complex disorder or group of disorders characterized by the onset of diffuse, often burning pain that typically is disproportionate to the precipitating stimulus" (Lindenfeld, 1998, p. 47). Clinical findings include abnormal blood flow to the extremity, hypersensitivity to cold or excessive sweating, abnormal reflex findings, and visual and palpable changes in superficial and deep tissues.

Treatment for reflex sympathetic dystrophy typically consists of prescribed oral corticosteroids to control global swelling and possibly a series of paravertebral blocks. Physical therapy is aimed at reducing edema and swelling, restoring normal range of motion, and strengthening relevant muscles to improve functional ability.

Other Complications

The unfortunate possibility of retearing any repaired site either spontaneously or through acute or chronic stress always exists. Possible neurological sequelae following surgery is another complication. Involvement of the sensory or motor nerves can also cause considerable dysfunction.

NUTRITIONAL CONSIDERATIONS

It is essential that patients closely monitor their nutritional status to make sure that they are taking in enough calories, water, vitamins, and minerals. Table 5.1 outlines general nutritional considerations to optimize healing. Preoperative evaluation of the patient's nutritional status and the treatment of low preoperative serum albumin levels have been definitively shown to correlate with improved outcome and decreased infection rates.

POSTOPERATIVE PSYCHOLOGICAL CONCERNS

Surgery can have both a positive and a negative impact on injured athletes. A successful surgery can provide relief of worry about the injury and its impact on future sports participation. At the same time, it can produce psychological distress. Most notably, after any type of invasive procedure, injured athletes will be physically drained and in significant pain, which can increase their emotional vulnerability. In addition, although the immediate and short-term threat of the surgery is behind them, they

TABLE 5.1
Nutritional Needs for Healing

	Rationale	Recommended	Sources
Water	Water is essential for healing an injury. It helps to decrease inflammation, therefore improving circulation and healing.	The average person requires a minimum of 5 cups of water a day. While recovering from surgery, try for at least 12 cups of fluid, preferably water.	
Vitamin C	Vitamin C functions in the making and maintaining of collagen, a protein that forms the base of your connective tissue. Connective tissue acts like cement between your cells, and it is found in high concentrations in the bones, teeth, tendons, muscles, skin, and joints. Vitamin C and collagen promote healing of wounds, bruises, and connective tissue injuries.	60–100 mg/day	Oranges, orange juice, strawberries, broccoli, cantaloupe, tomatoes and tomato juice, potatoes, cabbage, and greens
Vitamin E	Vitamin E is an antioxidant, which means it stabilizes cell membranes and protects cells and tissues from damage. Free-radical levels in the blood, which can damage the cells, increase during exercise, stress, injury, and surgery.	400 I.U. from natural sources	Wheat germ, and safflower and sunflower oil

(continues)

TABLE 5.1. *Continued.*

	Rationale	Recommended	Sources
Zinc	Zinc promotes healthy cell growth and development.	220 mg every other day	Oyster, turkey, liver, lima beans, and wheat germ
Magnesium	Magnesium helps to remove free radicals from the body and manufacture energy from carbohydrate, protein, and fat. A balance of calcium and magnesium is necessary to build healthy bone.	400 mg/day	Peanuts, bananas, beet greens, avocadoes, cashews, and whole grains

Note. Data are from *The Essential Guide to Vitamins and Minerals*, 1995, New York: HarperCollins. Copyright 1995 by HarperCollins.

are now faced with a protracted and uncomfortable recovery. Thus, the potential for emotional distress in the form of anxiety or depression is likely.

Psychological difficulties in patients affect them both emotionally and physically. Patients who are anxious or depressed have lower self-efficacy and lower expectations (Kurlowicz, 1998; Orbell, Johnston, Rowley, Espley, & Davey, 1998) and do not believe that they were fully healed (Szeverenyi et al., 1999). They also were found to experience more pain (Nelson, Zimmerman, Barnason, Nieveen, & Schmaderer, 1998). Patients suffering from emotional distress demonstrated less functional ability (Kurlowicz, 1998; Youmans, 1999), a lower perceived quality of life, and less adherence to recommended life changes (Kulik & Mahler, 1993).

There has been little discussion in the literature of why emotional difficulties have such a ubiquitous influence. We suggest several explanations drawing on the work of J. Taylor and Taylor (1997). Anxiety and depression directly interfere with immune activity and the healing process by inhibiting physiological contributors to recovery and creating a generalized sense of discomfort. Psychological distress also hurts patients' self-esteem and their belief that they can recover fully. These perceptions, in turn, produce an overall sense of dissatisfaction and lower perceived quality of life. Anxiety and depression also reduce patients' motivation to comply with rehabilitation recommendations, which results in slowed recovery and less-than-expected functional ability. What emerges is a cycle of negative thoughts, emotions, and behaviors that feed on one another to produce significant psychological, emotional, and physical obstacles to a full recovery.

Several strategies have been suggested to address patients' psychological distress. Self-hypnosis relaxation strategies have been advocated as a means of reducing the physical manifestations of anxiety. These techniques have been found to increase physical relaxation and reduce the need for pain medication (Ashton et al., 1997). Social support is the most common method recommended to combat emotional distress. It has been found to enhance self-esteem (Logsdon, Usui, Cronin, & Miracle, 1998), lower anxiety and depression (Kulik & Mahler, 1993), and produce higher self-efficacy and greater functional ability (Parent, 1997). The issues of relaxation training and social support are discussed further in Chapters 9 and 10.

As in the preoperative process, it is essential that the sports medicine team monitor and evaluate the psychological state of injured athletes after surgery. The presence of ongoing psychological distress (as described in Chapter 3) should alert the sports medicine team to take swift action to address the difficulties in the most timely and effective manner. Following the suggestions in Chapter 3 for identification and referral can ensure that injured athletes' psychological needs are addressed, facilitating their recovery.

SECTION III

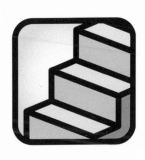

Rehabilitation

CHAPTER 6

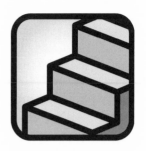

Recovery from Injury

The third phase of the injury management process shifts from the medical setting, where the physician is in charge and the focus is on the injury, to the physical therapy setting, where the physical therapist or athletic trainer takes over and the emphasis is on rehabilitation. This juncture presents a transition through which injured athletes move from being recipients of the diagnostic and surgical processes to being active participants in the rehabilitation process.

This step in the injury management process is another critical juncture for most injured athletes because they are faced with the prospect of having to endure a recovery process that is sometimes lengthy, is usually painful, and is always frustrating. It also signals a transition in their identity from injured athletes to recovering or rehabilitating athletes. In this new phase in the injury management process, injured athletes are in need of answers to the following questions:

- What can I expect during the course of my recovery?

- What are the common stages of recovery that I will go through?

- When will I be able to return to my sport?

- Will there be any long-term effects of my injury on my sports participation and other parts of my life?
- Can I expect a full recovery?

These are sensitive questions whose answers can have a significant impact on recovering athletes' attitudes toward their injury and the impending recovery process. Understanding these issues will influence recovering athletes' confidence in their ability to recover, their motivation to put in the effort required for a full recovery, the amount of stress they experience over whether they will recover fully, and their primary focus—past and negative or future and positive—as they initiate their rehabilitation program.

LENGTH OF REHABILITATION

A primary concern of injured athletes is how long it will take them to return to sport. The response to this question acts as injured athletes' first step in understanding the rehabilitation process and can influence their overall attitude toward their rehabilitation. Many rehabilitation professionals give a precise time frame, for example, 6 weeks for a knee arthroscopy. Offering such a specific time can create an expectation of recovery that may not be realistic for the particular situation. Rehabilitation and return to sport is not an exact science but instead is affected by many factors, including natural healing ability, effort put into rehabilitation, and complications that may arise. We recommend describing the usual range of duration for recovery from the particular type of injury, giving a typical upper and lower limit, then discussing what the patient can do to influence where in that range his or her recovery will fall. This approach ensures that injured athletes have a realistic perspective and a positive attitude toward rehabilitation, enhances their feelings of control over and responsibility for their recovery, and encourages them to be active participants in the rehabilitation process.

COURSE OF REHABILITATION

An important task for the sports medicine team is to make rehabilitation as familiar, predictable, and controllable as possible for injured athletes.

Fundamental to this task is imparting a realistic understanding of the course of rehabilitation. Injured athletes often hold inaccurate perceptions about how the rehabilitation process will progress, most notably, that recovery is a consistent process involving constant improvement. Yet, in reality, rehabilitation is a progressive, although unpredictable, process that has setbacks and plateaus. Beginning rehabilitation with unrealistic expectations can have a dramatic and damaging impact on an athlete's attitude, motivation, and feelings about recovery.

Understanding the course of rehabilitation will instill realistic perceptions and expectations about recovery, reduce the doubt and frustration in response to the normal ups and downs of rehabilitation, and foster a patient attitude that will allow healing and recovery to occur in its own time. Injured athletes will develop a perspective that will motivate them to adhere to their physical therapy program through the duration of rehabilitation. This understanding will enable them to respond positively to the many challenges and demands they will face as they progress through rehabilitation and return to sport.

An important component in understanding the course of rehabilitation is for patients to know the stages they will pass through toward full recovery. This awareness has several benefits. It provides the patients with a more clearly defined and predictable course of rehabilitation. It also increases their understanding of what occurs within each stage. Finally, particularly for injuries involving lengthy recoveries, it makes the rehabilitation process seem more manageable because, instead of one long and seemingly endless process, it now consists of shorter, more achievable stages.

STAGES OF REHABILITATION

There is no consensus on specific stages of rehabilitation (Shelbourne & Wilckens, 1990). However, a four-stage model has been suggested that is applicable to all injuries as a function of location, severity, and nature of injury: range of motion, strength, coordination, and return to sport (B. Fabrocini, personal communication, March 6, 1993; J. Taylor & Taylor, 1997). This model provides injured athletes with a better understanding of how they will progress through rehabilitation and what kinds of issues they will encounter along the way (see Table 6.1).

TABLE 6.1

Patient Education Guide: Stages of Physical Rehabilitation

Stage 1: Range of Motion

1. Goal: increase range of motion in injury area
2. Physical concern: pain
   a. Severe
   b. Unfamiliar
   c. Difficult to control
3. Psychological concern: helplessness
   a. Loss of confidence in injured area
   b. Worry about recovery from injury
   c. Negative focus on injury rather than positive focus on rehabilitation
   d. Drop in motivation to adhere to rehabilitation regimen
4. Recommendations
   a. Physical: learn about and use prescribed medication for pain management
   b. Psychological: learn about and use nondrug pain management, positive thinking, reorient away from injury and onto recovery, commitment to rehabilitation program

Stage 2: Strength

1. Goal: increase strength of injured area up to 80%
2. Physical concern: physical stress
   a. Initial postinjury physical demands placed on injured area
   b. Muscle bracing, generalized muscle tension, breathing difficulties
3. Psychological concern: psychological stress
   a. Worry about reaction of injured area to physical demands
   b. Doubt, anxiety, avoidance
4. Recommendations
   a. Physical: relaxation exercises, deep breathing, therapeutic massage
   b. Psychological: support and encouragement from sports medicine team, positive thinking, commitment to rehabilitation program

Stage 3: Coordination

1. Goal: integrate strength training with more complex muscle movement
2. Physical concern: limited performance
   a. Renewed use of injured area in "real world" situations
   b. Retraining coordination through the use of balance, agility, and speed exercises

(continues)

TABLE 6.1. *Continued.*

Stage 3: Coordination *Continued.*

3. Psychological concern: focus
   a. Easily distracted from effective execution of exercises
   b. Poor quality in rehabilitation exercises
4. Recommendations
   a. Physical: have patience with retraining of injured area, chart progress
   b. Psychological: pay close attention to instructions about proper execution of exercises, maintain "process focus" during exercises, gain confidence from progress

Stage 4: Return to Sport

1. Goal: return to full sport participation
2. Physical concern: stopping rehabilitation regimen prior to return to complete physical functioning
   a. Upward of 90% of full physical functioning
   b. Little pain and few physical limitations
   c. Perception that athlete is fully recovered
3. Psychological concern: confidence
   a. Poor performance upon initial return to sport
   b. Loss of confidence in ability to return to highest level
   c. Fear of reinjury
4. Recommendations
   a. Physical: maintain adherence to strict rehabilitation regimen until released by the sports medicine team
   b. Psychological: accept that performance will be poor upon initial return, rebuild confidence throughout recovery process, learn about causes and prevention of reinjury

Stage 1: Range of Motion

The goal of Stage 1 is to increase the range of motion at the injured area to a point where more functional aspects of rehabilitation can be concentrated on. Passive and active exercises that help the athletes regain their range of motion are the focus. The predominant issue for injured athletes in this first stage is the severe, unfamiliar, and seemingly uncontrollable pain they experience. Educating patients about different types of analgesic and nonanalgesic pain management is essential in Stage 1 so that the patients approach their pain with a constructive attitude (see Chapter 9).

Injured athletes' experiences with pain have psychological implications as well. Pain that is strong, unfamiliar, and uncontrollable will cause doubt and worry about the injury, erode confidence in the ability to recover, foster avoidance rather than adherence to physical therapy, and cause the athlete to focus on the negative aspects of the injury rather than on positive aspects of the rehabilitation.

Stage 2: Strength

As athletes enter the second stage, their range of motion should have returned to about 80% and will continue to improve (Davies & Zillmer, 2000). The goal of Stage 2 is to improve strength in the formerly injured area. Emphasis is placed on isometric, plyometric, and weight training exercises to rebuild strength lost because of the injury. Physical and psychological stress have the greatest impact on injured athletes in Stage 2. The physical stress occurs because this is the first time since the injury that the athlete has placed demands on the injured area, which failed the last time the athlete did so. So, naturally, this first test will cause doubt and uncertainty. This fear can result in psychological stress that results in breathing difficulties and muscle bracing, which will elevate pain and slow recovery.

This process can be facilitated by educating injured athletes about what they are likely to experience and how they can respond positively to the stress. They should also understand how physical and psychological stress can hinder rehabilitation and what tools they can use to minimize the negative effects (see Chapter 9).

Stage 3: Coordination

At the conclusion of Stage 2 there will be significant gains in strength around the injured area. Strength training will continue in Stage 3, but within a more integrated context that includes using more complex muscle movement to improve coordination. Exercises that address balance, agility, acceleration, and speed become the emphasis in rehabilitation as injured athletes move toward full functioning.

The primary psychological influence in Stage 3 is focus as injured athletes engage in complex physical therapy exercises that require special attention to proper execution. Without this "process focus," the quality of the rehabilitation exercises will be inadequate, and progress through

Stage 3 will be slowed. Injured athletes will benefit from very specific instructions about correct execution and focus on one or two keys that will ensure that they perform the exercises properly.

This stage of rehabilitation evolves into more "real world" use of the injured area as athletes move toward return to sport. Invariably, performance of these more realistic exercises will initially be well below preinjury levels. This comparison may be discouraging for injured athletes and hurt their confidence in their rehabilitation progress, which can lead to preoccupation with negative aspects of the injury and less attention to the progress they are making. Providing injured athletes with a realistic expectation of how they will advance through Stage 3 and giving them the tools to facilitate focus can allay their concerns and help them to maintain a positive focus on rehabilitation (see Chapter 8).

Stage 4: Return to Sport

Stage 4 marks the end of formal rehabilitation and athletes' return to participation in their sport. Although there is still injury-specific training to be done, physical testing will have shown that they have regained at least 90% of full physical functioning and are now ready to begin sport-specific training (Davies & Zillmer, 2000). However, contrary to most athletes' beliefs at this point, they are not fully recovered. Athletes' attitudes toward their rehabilitation early in their return to sport will often dictate whether they achieve the remaining 10% of functioning of the injured area.

As they enter Stage 4, athletes do not experience much pain and appear to have full functioning. Because of this high level of recovery, they may mistakenly interrupt their injury-specific training in the belief that it is no longer necessary. Yet, normal sport training does not usually provide for the full recovery needs of the once injured area, so the athletes do not continue to progress in these injury-specific areas and do not return to complete physical functioning. Without that full physical capability, athletes will not be able to return to their preinjury levels of performance. It is essential that the sports medicine team guard against this occurrence by emphasizing to injured athletes the need for strict adherence to all aspects of the rehabilitation regimen until they have clearly demonstrated a 100% restoration of functioning of all relevant dimensions as well as a return to preinjury performance.

The psychological focus in Stage 4 is on ensuring that athletes have the confidence they need to progressively build toward a successful return to sport. This issue is so important because many athletes return to full physical functioning yet do not perform up to preinjury level in training or competition owing to lack of confidence. Avoiding reinjury is the main concern as athletes return to sport. Educating them about how unlikely reinjury is and how the chances of reinjury can be reduced will allay concerns and enhance confidence.

The best means of building confidence is to develop a return-to-sport program that allows athletes to experience ongoing success while the injured area is tested in increasingly more difficult situations as the athletes progress through the return-to-sport process. With each positive experience with the rehabilitated area, athletes become more certain of its stability and health and more confident that it is capable of sustaining them under the renewed demands of intensive training and competition.

REHABILITATION SETBACKS

Setbacks are one of the most damaging experiences an athlete can have during rehabilitation. The message that setbacks usually send is that the athlete is not improving, but rather regressing. Perceptions about setbacks can have significant negative ramifications on all aspects of the rehabilitation process.

Setbacks, as they are usually perceived by injured athletes, have a negative impact on every psychological influence on rehabilitation, including confidence, motivation, stress, focus, and emotions. Yet, contrary to popular belief, setbacks are not necessarily negative and can, in fact, be positive. For setbacks not to be detrimental to an injured athlete's recovery, the athlete's attitude toward setbacks needs to be reshaped through education and understanding. J. Taylor and Taylor (1997) begin this reorientation by replacing the word *setback* with a phrase that they believe is more descriptive of what the experience is. They suggest that setbacks are a necessary part of the rehabilitation process and indicate that healing is occurring and provide information about the course of recovery. Setbacks can be seen as "rest periods" in preparation for another step in the healing process. The phrase *healing cycle* was created to give a more positive and precise description of those experiences (J. Taylor & Taylor, 1997). At a basic level, *healing cycle* will provide emotional relief because it does not carry the negative implications that *setback* does but rather suggests a normal, temporary phase of the healing process. Setbacks can also indicate whether the demands being placed on the athlete in rehabilitation are appropriate or if there is some physical problem that needs to be addressed.

There are specific healing cycles that are common to each stage of rehabilitation. A decline in range of motion and excessive swelling are typical in Stage 1, in which the injury is just beginning to heal and the body is not accustomed to the demands and pain of rehabilitation. Stage 2 healing cycles are marked by reduced strength as the body tries to protect itself from these new stressors. Typical healing cycles in the final two stages are swelling and pain as the body adapts to the newly integrated demands of strength and coordination training and the body's unfamiliarity with the intensity of sport training.

Although healing cycles are a normal part of the rehabilitation process, they should not simply be acknowledged and accepted. Rather, when healing cycles occur, they should be investigated and, if necessary, acted on to ensure that they do not slow the rehabilitation process. Healing cycles may indicate excessive efforts to rehabilitate by injured athletes. Some athletes are so motivated to recover that they act on the belief that more is better. This overadherence usually does more harm than good. A healing cycle is an attempt by the body to tell the athlete to slow down. A healing cycle may also suggest that the athlete is placing demands on the injured area that are too great for the present level of rehabilitation. Taking a step back in frequency or intensity can give the body time to adapt to the stresses and allow it to progress again.

Healing cycles may also signal a maladaptive response to noninjury-related stress. Physical indications may be tiredness, illness, and related injuries. Psychological stressors may include worry or frustration with the injury, depression or anxiety, or life stressors such as difficulties in school, work, or relationships.

Healing cycles are sources of information that the body is trying to convey to injured athletes. The message, most basically, is to make a change in some aspect of their rehabilitations or their lives. Common adjustments that injured athletes can make include modifying the frequency and intensity of physical therapy, changing specific components of the rehabilitation regimen, and providing more opportunities for rest and recuperation following demanding physical therapy efforts. Aside from physical therapy, possible changes are adjusting school or work schedules, resolving conflicts in relationships, and improving nutrition.

CHAPTER 7

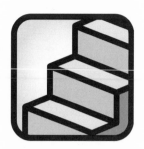

Physical Therapy

Physical therapy is the care and services provided by or under the direction and supervision of a physical therapist. Physical therapists provide services to patients who have impairments, functional limitations, disabilities, or changes in physical function and health status from injury, disease, or other causes ("Guide to Physical Therapy Practice," 1997). The goal of physical therapy in treating injured athletes is to assist the patient in fully rehabilitating from the injury and returning to the patient's previous level of activity.

PRACTICAL CONSIDERATIONS

Before recovering athletes explore the day-to-day details of what to expect during the rehabilitation process, they should first understand the practical concerns associated with physical therapy. This basic information will allow them to prepare effectively for the physical therapy program that lies ahead. There are many practical questions that recovering athletes should consider when selecting the therapy program for their needs.

111

- How do I find a physical therapist who specializes in rehabilitating my type of injury?

- What is my physical therapy going to cost me?

- How often will I need to go to physical therapy?

- How long will I attend physical therapy?

SELECTING A PHYSICAL THERAPIST

The rehabilitation process for many musculoskeletal injuries usually begins with a physician referral to physical therapy. The referral to physical therapy following evaluation by the physician typically contains orders for evaluation and treatment and may also include specific instructions from the physician regarding the type of physical therapy to be performed. Direct access to physical therapy—entry into physical therapy without a physician referral—is legal in most states but not common, because insurance carriers require a physician referral to process claims and pay for physical therapy services.

Referrals to physical therapy most often come from medical doctors but may come from doctors of osteopathic medicine, chiropractors, podiatrists, and dentists. The physical therapy referral includes the patient's diagnosis and the frequency and duration of physical therapy. The referral to a physical therapy clinic is usually based on the familiarity of the referring physician with the physical therapist. The physical therapist and physician should have a working relationship, especially in postoperative rehabilitation referrals, because knowledge of the specific techniques and rehabilitation goals and concepts of the surgeon is critically important. Although there are many physical therapy offices throughout the United States, obtaining a referral to a therapist who has an established specialty and competence in treating the specific injury, disease process, or disability is also important.

The American Physical Therapy Association (APTA) is the national organization representing physical therapists and has programs for certifying therapists in areas of specialization. These areas of specialization include cardiopulmonary, clinical, electrophysical, geriatric, neurologic, orthopedic, pediatric, and sports physical therapy. Selecting a licensed physical therapist ensures that the therapist has graduated from an accredited educational program in physical therapy and has passed the national licensure examination. Choosing a physical therapist who is not only licensed but also specializes in treating the athlete's specific injury is recommended. Therapists who have obtained a specialization are recognized by using designated initials after their name. Information about physical therapists and their qualifications, as well as information regarding specialists in specific geographic locations, can be obtained by contacting the American Physical Therapy Association (111 North Fairfax St., Alexandria, VA 22314; tel: 800/999-APTA; www.apta.org). As with selecting other medical professionals, careful selection of the physical therapist will help to ensure the highest level of care for the specific injury.

COST OF PHYSICAL THERAPY

The cost of physical therapy will vary, according to geographic location, type of physical therapy required, and type of rehabilitation center used. Patients should take an active role in educating themselves about costs, because it is ultimately both the patient's and the insurance company's responsibility for covering the cost of the physical therapy services. It is best for the patients to contact their insurance company directly regarding the exact benefits and limitations of their health plan. Examples of limitations that insurance companies place on treatment include the number of treatments in a calendar year, the number of treatments with or without authorization, and the number of treatments per diagnosis. Additionally, payment for physical therapy services often depends on where the patient goes for physical therapy, because insurance companies often contract with a network of providers of physical therapy, and when a patient chooses from within this network, the insurance company provides greater coverage for the cost of physical therapy care.

Another person who can be contacted regarding the cost of physical therapy is the office manager of the physical therapy clinic the patient will use. These individuals have specialized training in the reimbursement procedures of many insurance companies and can provide an estimate of the approximate cost of physical therapy as well as an estimate of the patient's financial responsibility for the physical therapy. Obtaining this specific information prior to initiating physical therapy ensures that both the patient and the physical therapy provider are aware of the financial responsibilities for the treatments.

Charges for most physical therapy services are based on procedure or number of procedures provided. For example, many patients receive modalities such as electrical stimulation, ultrasound, or iontophoresis to decrease pain and inflammation during the early stages of rehabilitation. Each procedure carries a specific charge. Additional procedures, such as exercise, stretching, and testing and evaluation, are often billed according to the amount of time involved. Some of these procedures, such as therapeutic exercise, manual therapy, and evaluation, often carry a higher charge because greater levels of supervision and physical therapist involvement are required.

FREQUENCY OF PHYSICAL THERAPY

The frequency of physical therapy varies significantly according to type of injury, surgical procedure performed, and rehabilitation regimen prescribed. Additionally, there have been significant changes in recent years in the number of treatments allowed for and covered by insurance companies for certain diagnoses. Accordingly, it is difficult to give anything more than estimates or trends for frequency of physical therapy treatment.

Typical frequency of physical therapy treatment ranges from as little as once a week to as often as daily. In today's managed care environment, the number of patients seen daily in outpatient rehabilitation centers for musculoskeletal diagnoses is very small. Indications for daily treatments for a musculoskeletal injury include extreme pain, swelling, loss of range of motion, and weakness. Examples of such injuries are a severe thigh contusion or an anterior cruciate ligament (ACL) reconstruction followed by severe swelling, loss of motion, and inability to actively contract the musculature around the knee volitionally. Even with these severe injuries, daily care would not continue for very long, owing to limitations in the number of visits allowed for such an injury as well as other provider limitations.

Many physical therapy referrals call for treatment sessions two to three times per week. This is common for most musculoskeletal diagnoses seen in outpatient rehabilitation clinics. An every-other-day treatment schedule allows for a day of recovery between sessions but requires home exercise and active patient participation in the rehabilitation program. As rehabilitation continues, the frequency of formal physical therapy care decreases from about three times a week to once a week or every other week. This allows for extended monitoring of patient signs and symptoms as well as advancement of home exercise programming and objective testing. With the decrease in the number of formal physical therapy visits, it is essential that the patient be committed to the home exercise instructions given by the therapist to ensure continued progress toward recovery. Failure to perform home-based exercise and rehabilitation programming can severely jeopardize improvement and increases the need for extended formal physical therapy programming.

DURATION OF PHYSICAL THERAPY

The duration of physical therapy also varies widely according to type of injury, surgical procedure, and rehabilitation regimen. Examples of typical postoperative rehabilitation durations include 4–6 weeks for knee arthroscopy, 6–8 weeks for shoulder arthroscopy for partial rotator cuff tears, and 12 weeks for open rotator cuff repair, arthroscopic and open Bankart reconstructions, and ACL reconstructions. These are simply clinical estimates, and further rehabilitation through home exercise and interval return-to-sport programs is required in many cases. Estimated duration of physical therapy for common musculoskeletal diagnoses seen in a sports medicine program is shown in Table 7.1. These data were compiled from more than 1,700 cases in an outpatient orthopedic and sports medicine clinic in the middle to late 1980s (Derscheid & Feiring, 1987). More specific information regarding the estimated frequency and duration of the patient's physical therapy can be obtained by consulting with the referring physician and the physical therapist.

TABLE 7.1
Frequency and Duration of Physical Therapy
for Various Musculoskeletal Diagnoses

Injury/Surgery	Treatment Frequencies	Duration (weeks)
ACL reconstruction	39	15.5
Medial meniscectomy	15	6.0
Chondromalacia	14	3.5
Lateral ankle sprain	9	3.5
Plantarfasciitis	9	3.5
Shoulder impingement	14	6.0
Rotator cuff tendonosis	14	6.0
Lateral epicondylitis	8	3.5
Lumbar sprain	6	2.5

PHYSICAL THERAPY PROGRAM

The physical therapy phase of injury management is perhaps the most difficult, because rehabilitation is an intensive and oftentimes complicated process that places physical, psychological, emotional, and logistical demands on injured athletes. Rehabilitating athletes are now faced with the unfamiliarity and unpredictability of what may appear to them to be a distant and difficult goal to achieve, namely, a timely and successful recovery and return to sport. As athletes make the transition from perceiving themselves as damaged to seeing themselves as recovering, they can become overwhelmed with the demands they must face in physical therapy. In facing these demands, rehabilitating athletes can benefit greatly from answers to the following questions:

- What are the specific components of my physical therapy program?
- What are my responsibilities in physical therapy?
- What goals should I set for my rehabilitation?
- How can I stay in shape and not fall behind in my sport?

The answers to these questions will enable recovering athletes to view rehabilitation as both manageable and achievable. This knowledge will allow them not only to play an active part in their physical therapy but also to take on a leading role in their rehabilitation and return to sport.

COMPONENTS OF THE PHYSICAL THERAPY PROGRAM

Important components of a comprehensive physical therapy program include an initial evaluation, physical therapy treatments, a home exercise program, an interval return-to-sport program, and a discharge evaluation.

- *Initial Evaluation.* The most critical aspect of the physical therapy program is the initial evaluation, during which the therapist gains the information required to successfully treat the patient. The initial evaluation usually begins with the therapist's obtaining a thorough history, by asking specific questions regarding the patient's current musculoskeletal status, general medical health, past history of injury, and both work and sport requirements. To ensure an effective physical therapy program, the patient must provide accurate and detailed information during this evaluation. In taking a comprehensive history, the physical therapist can use the same form that the sports medicine physician uses to record the patient's history (see Figure 1.1).

After taking the patient's history, the therapist performs objective testing and measurement of critically important physical parameters such as posture and stance, anthropometric girths to detect swelling or muscular atrophy, muscular strength, range of motion, and motor and sensory function. The therapist also conducts a series of joint-specific tests to assess the competency of structures around joints such as menisci, ligaments, and tendons as well as the stability and integrity of the joint surfaces. These tests help the therapist to better understand the extent of the injury and to determine which structures require rehabilitation. The initial evaluation process can take as long as 1 hour and requires one-on-one interaction with the therapist. Because initial entry paperwork and insurance information are processed prior to the initial evaluation, and because this visit is usually combined with a treatment, it is typically the longest visit in the physical therapy program.

• *Physical Therapy Treatments.* Physical therapy treatments following the patient's first visit typically involve use of modalities to control pain and encourage healing of the injured structures as well as manual therapy such as mobilization of the joints and passive stretching to improve range of motion. Additional therapeutic exercise is usually employed in varying amounts according to the patient's tolerance for pain, the extent of injury, and the stage of rehabilitation.

Exercise-based therapy is widely used in the United States and is the largest component of rehabilitation. Typical time duration of a treatment of physical therapy ranges from as little as 45 minutes to several hours, depending on the amount of general and sport-specific conditioning that is combined with the injury-specific treatment. As the patient progresses, the duration of each visit typically increases, owing to the heavy reliance on therapeutic exercise.

• *Home Exercise Program.* Formulating and administering a home exercise program is an important component of the physical therapy regimen. The home program is designed to reinforce the treatment program that is performed in the clinic and to complement the rehabilitation program, range-of-motion exercises, and stretching that are performed under the guidance of the therapist. The home program is not meant to act as a substitute for formal physical therapy and supervised care, but it is an important part of the therapy program and demands commitment and compliance from the patient. To ensure proper home exercise performance, therapists should provide patients with detailed descriptions and demonstrations of all exercises and procedures. Figure 7.1 shows a sample home exercise program for tennis elbow.

(*text continues on p. 120*)

LATERAL EPICONDYLITIS (TENNIS ELBOW) HOME PROGRAM

- Posture, posture, posture—always practice good mechanics when standing, sitting, lifting, etc. Be especially aware if you sit for long periods of time. Take regular breaks and get up and change positions so your shoulders do not fall into poor posture. This will also make you rely on your stronger arm and shoulder muscles to do more of the work than your weaker elbow muscles.

- Ice the forearm and elbow for 10–15 minutes 3–5 times a day. Ice massage (10 mm) or ice bags will both work fine. Ice massage may be best performed by freezing water in a paper cup, then peeling off the top half of the paper, holding the base of the cup and then pressing the ice onto the injured area in a circular fashion.

- A wrist splint that holds the wrist in a neutral position may be used for sleeping and any repetitive grasping or gripping activities. This rests the injured tendon.

- Regularly throughout the day (3–5 times):

    Stretch the wrist and forearm by extending the arm and grasping the fingertips and slowly bring them down and underneath the forearm. Hold 15 seconds. Repeat 2 times in 3 different positions of arm rotation.

    Stretch the thumb and wrist by extending the arm, resting it on a table with the palm facing inward; grasp the thumb and hand with your opposite hand and slowly bend in a direction opposite the thumb. Hold 15 seconds. Repeat 3 times.

    Stretch the chest by lightly grasping a doorjamb with your fingers just below shoulder height, relax your arm and slowly rotate your body away from your arm. Hold 15 seconds. Repeat 3 times.

    Keep your neck loose by bending it from side to side 5 times and then rotate one way then the other 5 times.

- Once a day, arm supported on a table, palm facing up and with the elbow bent, slowly flex or curl up a light weight with your wrist and hand, then lower. The lowering phase should be twice as long as the lifting/curling. Work up to 2 sets of 20 repetitions.

- Rotator cuff program: Stand up straight with a resisted band wrapped around the wrist, the elbow bent, and a pillow or folded towel under the arm. Rotate the arm inward against the band and then rotate out. Do 2 sets of 20–30 repetitions. Repeat the same, rotating outward against the band.

ACL HOME EXERCISE PROGRAM

Always precede any workout routine with some form of cardio warm-up. Stationary bike, elliptical, stair machine, and NordicTrak are great options. Can also do

(continues)

Figure 7.1. Sample home exercise programs.

circuit cardio with 3 different machines at higher intensity and shorter periods for your set time and without resting in between.

Sample: Stationary bike @ 90–110 RPMs for 10 minutes; Elliptical machine working at 75% intensity for 10 minutes

Treadmill walking with a 5%–7% grade with arm swing for 10 minutes

Stretching: Hold each for 20–30 seconds and repeat 3 times each:

- Hamstrings while either standing and heel on a step and back straight leaning forward, or seated with heel on another chair/bench and sitting up straight
- Calves with forefoot on a rolled-up towel and leg straight; slowly lean forward
- Flexion/thigh while seated and bringing your leg toward you until it stretches

Monday / Wednesday / Friday

- Weight machines: 1 set with both legs and 1 set with one leg:

    Leg press

    Hamstrings

    Abduction/adduction

    Calf machine or raises

- Physio ball rolls: Lying on back with back of lower legs on ball, lift hips and flex and extend legs 2 sets of 20–30 repetitions
- Single-leg balance: On a folded pillow or couple of towels, vary the position of knee bend and hold each position for 15–30 seconds
- Lunge stepping–down a hallway, weight through the heel of the front foot for 1–2 minutes
- Crunches: 3 sets to fatigue, focusing on "drawing in" on the abdominals

Tuesday / Thursday / Saturday

- Squats/double knee bends: Feet shoulder distance apart, physio ball held out in front of you, no pause on the way up or down. One set of 1–3 minutes. Perform a second set with the use of the resistance cable (red).
- Calf raises: On the ground without holding on to anything, with both legs and then with one leg. Two sets to fatigue.
- Standing toe curls: Equal weight on both feet, curl toes under feet as if lightly rolling to the outside of your feet. Hold 5 seconds. Repeat 10 times.

(continues)

Figure 7.1. *Continued.*

Tuesday / Thursday / Saturday Continued.

- Single leg forward step-ups: Weight through the heel of the front foot and not pushing up with the rear foot. Hips level and smooth motion. Two sets of 1–2 minutes.

- Hamstring bridging: Both heels on a physio ball and knees bent, lift and lower hips without resting hips on ground. Two sets of 30–40 repetitions.

- Resistance cable squats: With belt, perform squats while left side to the cable and then with right side. One set of each for 1–2 minutes.

- Single-leg balance: Standing on a step with other leg stabilized and hanging off the side in a tuck position with stable hips.

Finish program with a light stretching routine and ice if possible.

Figure 7.1. *Continued.*

- *Interval Return-to-Sport Program.* As the patient comes to the end of the formal rehabilitation program and nears his or her return to sport participation, the therapist will place the patient on an interval return-to-sport program. The details of this program are discussed in Chapter 11 and in Appendixes A and B. The interval return-to-sport program plays an important role in bridging the gap between the physical therapy program and the athlete's full return to sport.

- *Discharge Evaluation.* Prior to discharging the patient from formal physical therapy, the therapist usually reassesses the final range-of-motion and strength levels as well as other functional and joint-specific measures that were tested during the initial evaluation. The therapist than updates the home exercise program and incorporates additional exercises to maintain or further develop strength and range of motion. Additionally, specific instructions regarding warming up and cooling down and return-to-sport functioning are included. These elements ensure that all aspects of the rehabilitation are evaluated and the continued presence of deficits or disabilities are highlighted and emphasized in the home postrehabilitation exercise training programs to ameliorate them and prevent further injury or reinjury.

PATIENT RESPONSIBILITIES FOR PHYSICAL THERAPY

From the start to the conclusion of a physical therapy program, the patient has several important responsibilities. The first lies in learning about the practical aspects of physical therapy. It is the patient's responsibility to obtain as much information as possible about the therapist and the clinic to ensure that they are reputable and good choices for rehabilitation. It is also the patient's responsibility to learn about the financial issues related to rehabilitation. In general, an informed patient gets more out of physical therapy than one who takes little or no interest or responsibility in the rehabilitation process.

The patient must also initiate and persist in physical therapy efforts. Patients who take ownership in their rehabilitation largely determine the speed and effectiveness of their recovery and return to sport. This commitment translates into total compliance with attendance at scheduled physical therapy sessions, observance of exercise and activity restrictions, and adherence to home exercise instructions.

REHABILITATION GOAL SETTING

Goal setting is a widely advocated strategy for providing direction and impetus in sports (Feltz, 1986; Fisher, Mullins, & Frye, 1993; Grove & Gordon, 1992). Injured athletes and rehabilitation professionals agree that rehabilitation goals can encourage motivation and bolster adherence to the physical therapy process (Brewer, Jeffers, Petitpas, & Van Raalte, 1994; Duda, Smart, & Tappe, 1989; Ievleva & Orlick, 1991). Goal setting offers injured athletes a "road map" to their desired destination—a timely and effective recovery. Goals help injured athletes to understand what they need to do during physical therapy to maximize their rehabilitation efforts. Goals also increase athletes' sense of familiarity, predictability, and control over their recoveries. Fostering these perceptions has the additional effect of improving confidence, lowering stress, and helping maintain a positive and constructive focus.

Goal setting offers injured athletes clear and specific steps that lead to complete recovery. These objectives will discourage them from trying to rush the healing process or avoid aspects of rehabilitation that are important. Goals provide the means for directing injured athletes' motivation in a productive way. Simply put, goals show injured athletes what they need to do to recover and return to sport in the fastest and most effective way possible.

The best way to use goals to facilitate the injury management process is to create an organized rehabilitation goal-setting program. This program offers injured athletes clearly defined goals for every area they need to address for a successful recovery. It places the goals in the most effective format and details the particular means by which the goals will be achieved.

Physical and Psychological Rehabilitation Goals

Goals should be created for each physical dimension associated with recovery from the injury, including range of motion, strength, stability, stamina, and flexibility. Goals for each of these areas should specify the physical component to be addressed, the specific area to be worked on, the final outcome for the parameter, and the way in which the goal will be achieved.

Developing a goal-setting program starts with discussions between the rehabilitation professional and the injured athlete about the physical dimensions that are relevant for the athlete's individualized rehabilitation program. This dialogue will increase the athlete's understanding of the role that each element plays in the overall rehabilitation program. It also allows the athlete to be an informed and active participant in developing the rehabilitation goal-setting program.

Injured athletes should view psychological rehabilitation in the same way that they do physical rehabilitation: For a complete recovery to occur, psychological damage must be rehabilitated in much the same manner as the physical injury. Injured athletes should set a series of goals for psychological issues that affect rehabilitation and return to sport, including confidence, motivation, stress, and focus.

Performance Goals

If injured athletes want to minimize the deterioration of their sport-specific abilities, these areas must be a part of their rehabilitation goal-setting program. Without these goals, performance issues are often relegated to a lower priority or neglected altogether during rehabilitation. Performance issues should be addressed by developing a sport training program to accompany the physical therapy program. Injured athletes can identify the areas on which they want to work, decide what their ultimate goals in those areas are, and specify how they will work toward the goals.

Technical and tactical skills are the first area for which performance goals should be set. Injured athletes should ask themselves, "What technical and tactical skills do I need to maintain or improve to make me a better athlete upon my return to sport?" Then they can ask, "What do I need to do during my rehabilitation to work on those skills?" The answers to these questions will provide the necessary information for setting appropriate performance goals for technique and tactics.

Physical conditioning is another area in which injured athletes can make improvements during rehabilitation. A conditioning program that works around the injury can enable athletes to return to sport in better shape than they were prior to the injury. Establishing specific physical conditioning goals will provide injured athletes with a focus and direction in their non–injury-related physical training during the healing process. This approach also has psychological advantages: It builds confidence, relieves stress, directs focus positively, and reassures athletes that they are furthering their athletic development during rehabilitation.

Rehabilitation also offers injured athletes the opportunity to develop their mental skills on two levels. First, psychological rehabilitation can augment many aspects of the recovery process by addressing issues that can either facilitate or interfere with healing and rehabilitation, for example, the athlete's attitude. Second, injured athletes can use this time to identify and work on psychological traits that have hampered past performances, for instance, anxiety or lack of confidence. Much like physical conditioning, setting and achieving goals to enhance mental aspects of performance will allow injured athletes to return to sport more mentally prepared than before their injury. Common mental skills that injured athletes can incorporate into their performance goals include confidence building, muscle relaxation, focusing techniques, precompetition routines, and sport imagery.

Return-to-sport goals are critical for a successful transition from rehabilitation to return to sport. With the end of the injury management process in sight, two responses can interfere with its completion. First, athletes may be overzealous in their desire to return to competition. This excessive enthusiasm can lead to slowed rather than accelerated recovery. Return-to-sport goals help athletes to test their expectations and moderate their desire to return by setting clear objectives that will steadily lead them to their final goal of a timely and effective return to sport. Second, athletes may have unrealistic expectations about how they will perform when they first begin playing again. When they do not perform up to expectations right stage goals should use objective measures to assess progress in key physical areas. Psychological stage goals can also be established as a means of assisting injured athletes in achieving their psychological recovery goals. Psychological stage goals focus on specific psychological factors that need to be addressed. Athletes can choose one or two psychological areas to work on in each stage. For example, goals related to motivation and pain management may be the emphasis in the first stage, when rehabilitation is most difficult and painful, whereas in the fourth stage, confidence and focus may be stressed in preparation for return to sport.

Performance stage goals include sport-specific issues such as physical conditioning and technical improvement. We recommend that physical conditioning be the focus in the early stages of rehabilitation, followed by technical work and tactical development, because it takes more time to make gains in physical fitness than in technical or tactical work.

Daily Goals

Daily goals may be the most important objectives to establish—it is one thing for injured athletes to know where they are going, but it is another thing to know how to get there. Daily goals tell injured athletes what they need to accomplish each day in physical therapy to achieve their stage and recovery goals. Daily goals provide both the direction and focus for each day's physical therapy efforts. Daily goals identify the type, quantity, and purpose of exercises and modalities injured athletes need to engage in during their physical therapy sessions.

Daily goals are not usually incorporated into the formal rehabilitation goal-setting program, because daily physical therapy activities depend largely on the level of progress injured athletes are making and how they feel at that point in their physical therapy program. Instead, daily goals are set at the end of the previous day's session or just before the start of a new one. Even when they are set just prior to physical therapy, they should still be clearly and tangibly stated and connected to injured athletes' stage and recovery goals.

Lifestyle Goals

One of the most common complaints of injured athletes undergoing rehabilitation is that they are much more tired than usual. Unfortunately, few injured athletes realize the physical toll that rehabilitation takes on their overall life. Yet, not only does rehabilitation affect their daily life, but their lifestyle also can either facilitate or interfere with their recoveries.

Lifestyle issues such as sleep, diet, alcohol or drug use, relationships, work, and school can all help or hurt their rehabilitation.

Injured athletes should examine their lifestyle and identify the areas that are affecting their recovery positively or negatively. Then, if certain areas are holding them back, they can make adjustments in their lifestyle so that all aspects of their life are working together toward a timely and successful recovery.

Developing a Rehabilitation Goal-Setting Program

Developing a rehabilitation goal-setting program is an excellent opportunity to show injured athletes that their recovery is a coordinated effort between themselves and members of the sports medicine team. Early in the rehabilitation process, injured athletes can be educated about the value and purpose of goal setting. They can then learn about the specific aspects of goal setting, including the types of goals and the guidelines for setting goals. Then, in collaboration with members of the sports medicine team, they can create recovery, stage, and lifestyle goals that will foster their rehabilitation efforts. A rehabilitation goal-setting form that can be used to specify goals is shown in Figure 7.2.

When injured athletes have completed their rehabilitation goal-setting program, they and the sports medicine team can sign a rehabilitation contract (see Figure 7.3). A formalized contract clarifies the responsibilities of all parties involved in the rehabilitation and enhances injured athletes' commitment to their goals and compliance with the rehabilitation program. The cooperative nature of the contract acts to build trust between injured athletes and the sports medicine team and encourages in the athletes a feeling of support and coordinated effort in working toward their goals.

MAINTAINING GENERAL PHYSICAL FITNESS

Another important component of a comprehensive physical therapy program for injured athletes is an alternative exercise regimen to help them maintain and build on their general physical fitness and their

(*text continues on p. 132*)

REHABILITATION GOAL-SETTING PROGRAM

Directions. In the tables below, set the Recovery, Stage, and Lifestyle goals for
your rehabilitation. Follow the goal guidelines described [in the text] to ensure
that you set the most effective goals possible.

Recovery Goals

Physical	Psychological	Performance

(continues)

Figure 7.2. Rehabilitation Goal-Setting Program. *Note.* From *Psychological Approaches to Sports Injury Rehabilitation* (pp. 139–141), by J. Taylor and S. Taylor, 1997, Austin, TX: PRO-ED. Copyright 1997 by PRO-ED, Inc. Reprinted with permission.

		Stage Goals	
	Physical	*Psychological*	*Performance*
Stage 1			
Goal #1			
method			
Goal #2			
method			
Stage 2			
Goal #1			
method			
Goal #2			
method			
Stage 3			
Goal #1			
method			
Goal #2			
method			
Stage 4			
Goal #1			
method			
Goal #2			
method			

(continues)

Figure 7.2. *Continued.*

Lifestyle Goals

Sleep	Diet	Relationships	Work/School	Other

Figure 7.2. *Continued.*

REHABILITATION CONTRACT

Injured Athlete

I, _____, agree to diligently fulfill my responsibilities in the rehabilitation of my injury. These responsibilities include

1. Taking full control of all aspects of my rehabilitation
2. Precise adherence to the rehabilitation program designed for me
3. Attendance at all scheduled physical therapy sessions
4. Completion of all exercises outside of the rehabilitation facility
5. Full effort, focus, and intensity in all aspects of my rehabilitation regimen
6. Consistent pursuit of the goals I set in my rehabilitation goal setting program
7. Developing psychological areas that impact my recovery and return to sport
8. Improving myself as an athlete during rehabilitation
9. Seeking out assistance from others when difficulties arise

Rehabilitation Professional

I, _____, agree to diligently fulfill my responsibilities as the rehabilitation professional in the rehabilitation of _____'s injury. These responsibilities include

1. Designing an individualized rehabilitation program for the injured athlete
2. Educating the athlete about all relevant aspects of the rehabilitation process
3. Helping to establish a series of goals that will progressively lead to full recovery and return to sport
4. Creating a rehabilitation team with other relevant professionals
5. Being sensitive and responsive to psychological and emotional needs
6. Assisting the athlete in overcoming physical and psychological obstacles that may arise during rehabilitation
7. Providing the athlete with the information and skills to facilitate physical, psychological, and performance contributors to a successful return to sport

_____	_____
Athlete	Date
_____	_____
Professional	Date

Figure 7.3. Rehabilitation Contract. *Note.* From *Psychological Approaches to Sports Injury Rehabilitation* (p. 142), by J. Taylor and S. Taylor, 1997, Austin, TX: PRO-ED. Copyright 1997 by PRO-ED, Inc. Reprinted with permission.

sport-specific proficiency. When athletes suffer a serious injury, they often cease training or cut back considerably. For example, a runner who injures a knee cannot, in most cases, continue to maintain the same level of cardiovascular fitness. Because it is imperative, however, that cardiovascular capacity be maintained during rehabilitation, the runner might decide to develop a swimming regimen for that purpose.

In addition, specific programming geared at maintaining and developing sport-specific muscular strength, endurance, and flexibility can be incorporated into the physical therapy program. For example, a tennis player with an injured shoulder can almost always perform exercises for the forearm and wrist early in the rehabilitation program without harming the shoulder. Wrist and forearm strengthening would improve distal strength and endurance levels while the shoulder is healing and undergoing rehabilitation.

Injured athletes gain many physical and psychological benefits by maintaining overall fitness during rehabilitation. Changes in body composition—gaining or losing weight—due to inactivity can be prevented. Return to sport can be facilitated for athletes at a high level of general physical conditioning when they complete their rehabilitation. Athletes who reenter their sport in excellent physical condition are also more mentally prepared and have greater confidence about returning to their preinjury level of performance.

CHAPTER 8

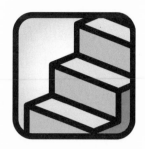

Psychological Concerns in Rehabilitation

The goal of rehabilitation is to fully heal the injured area and allow athletes to return to their sport physically prepared to perform at or above their preinjury level. Therefore, physical therapy is the primary focus of the rehabilitation process. Because of this, perhaps the most neglected aspect of rehabilitation is the psychological recovery from the injury. Although rehabilitation professionals and athletes alike attest to the psychological and emotional challenges of an injury, little attention is paid to healing the psychological "muscles" that sustain damage from the physical injury. Discussing the following concerns can help injured athletes understand and surmount the psychological ramifications of physical injury:

- How do I keep from losing confidence in my healing and in myself as an athlete?

- How do I stay motivated during my long and painful rehabilitation?

- How do I keep from getting overstressed by the rehabilitation process?

- How do I focus on the positive aspects of my rehabilitation rather than the negative aspects of my injury?

- What mental stratagems can I use to facilitate my rehabilitation?

The quality and extent of rehabilitation achieved by injured athletes depends on their attitude toward physical therapy. The reality is that physical therapy can be an uncomfortable, repetitious, and tedious experience. It is difficult for injured athletes to maintain the level of physical therapy necessary to have a timely and effective recovery. Injured athletes' ability to sustain the requisite effort depends on their ability to maintain an attitude of confidence, motivation, and focus. Providing them with the tools to encourage this attitude will pay important dividends at the conclusion of rehabilitation.

CONFIDENCE IN REHABILITATION

The single most influential psychological determinant of the ultimate outcome of the injury management process is how strongly the athletes believe that they can complete rehabilitation and return to their sport. Injured athletes may be physically able to recover fully, but if they lack the confidence to do so, the level of rehabilitation will be insufficient to ensure a complete recovery. Confidence is so important because it directly influences injured athletes' efforts during rehabilitation and also affects other psychological contributors to recovery.

J. Taylor and Taylor (1997) have suggested that confidence can produce either a negative vicious cycle or a positive upward spiral in rehabilitation. The vicious cycle starts with low confidence, which produces negative self-talk; negative emotions such as anger, depression, and frustration; physical stress; an interfering focus; and low motivation. The result of the vicious cycle is a poor-quality rehabilitation and an incomplete recovery. In contrast, the upward spiral begins with high confidence, which leads to positive self-talk, positive emotions, a relaxed physical state, a facilitating focus, and high motivation. The outcome of the upward spiral is a high-quality rehabilitation and a timely and effective recovery.

Research provides support for this position. For example, injured athletes tend to focus on the negative aspects of the injury rather than on positive elements of the rehabilitation (Weiss & Troxel, 1986). Additionally, athletic trainers have indicated that positive attitude is an important characteristic differentiating athletes who cope successfully from those who cope less successfully with an injury (Wiese, Weiss, & Yukelson, 1991). The study showed that fostering positive self-talk is a useful tool for enhancing coping among injured athletes. Additional research also supports the notion that confidence directly affects rehabilitation: Injured athletes who believe in their rehabilitation programs demonstrate greater adherence (Duda, Smart, & Tappe, 1989).

Four Levels of Rehabilitation Confidence

Rehabilitation confidence is more than just the degree to which injured athletes believe they can rehabilitate their injury and return to their sport. It is a multidimensional factor that affects many parts of the injury management process (see Table 8.1).

Program Confidence

The foundation of confidence for injured athletes lies in how strongly they believe that their rehabilitation program will enable them to have a complete recovery. Program confidence can be developed in several ways. Initially, it comes from the rehabilitation staff. If they believe in the program, the injured athletes with whom they work are likely to do so as well. Also, educating patients about their rehabilitation program will increase its predictability and the patients' sense of control, which, in turn, will enhance their confidence in the program. The rehabilitation staff can also show injured athletes scientific research documenting the rehabilitation program's effectiveness and introduce them to athletes who had similar injuries, were on comparable programs, and made full recoveries.

Adherence Confidence

Perhaps the most challenging form of rehabilitation confidence involves how strongly injured athletes believe that they can adhere to their rehabilitation program. Often, the path to rehabilitation is long, demanding, and painful. It is natural that injured athletes will question whether they can complete such an arduous journey. Developing adherence confidence involves a gradual process of becoming familiar with rehabilitation and physical therapy and developing realistic, experience-based perceptions, expectations, and goals about the rehabilitation process.

TABLE 8.1

Developing the Four Levels of Confidence

Level of Confidence	Development Strategy
Program Confidence	Be a confident role model about program effectiveness
	Increase familiarity, predictability, and control
	Ensure rehabilitation education
	Provide scientific and athletic evidence of program effectiveness
Adherence Confidence	Show similarity between sport and rehabilitation skills
	Set small, manageable goals
	Increase understanding of rehabilitation
Physical Confidence	Ensure recognition of healing and positive response to demands of rehabilitation
	Maintain rigorous physical-conditioning program
	Identify confident role models
	Keep good attitude toward ups and downs of rehabilitation
	Use psychological rehabilitation techniques
Return-to-Sport Confidence	Perception that rehabilitation has been successfully completed
	Belief that injury is fully healed
	Sound level of overall physical conditioning
	Technique and tactics have been maintained
	Positive levels of confidence, motivation, anxiety, and focus
	Realistic and patient attitude about progression from initial training to return to competition

Note. From *Psychological Approaches to Sports Injury Rehabilitation* (p. 102), by J. Taylor and S. Taylor, 1997, Austin, TX: PRO-ED. Copyright 1997 by PRO-ED, Inc. Reprinted with permission.

Adherence rehabilitation can also be facilitated by introducing injured athletes to the notion that "rehabilitation is athletic performance." If they can make this connection, they will see that they already possess many of the skills to successfully complete rehabilitation, including determination, focus, and the ability to overcome obstacles. Adherence confidence can also be fostered by giving injured athletes small, manageable goals that they can achieve. For example, it may be difficult for injured athletes to believe that they can make it through the entire rehabilitation process, but they can have confidence that they can adhere to their program for the next week. With incremental progress, injured athletes will be encouraged by increased familiarity with the rehabilitation process, improved functioning, and decreased pain, thereby creating an upward spiral of adherence confidence.

Physical Confidence

Physical confidence relates to injured athletes' belief that the damaged area can withstand the demands of performance when they return to sport. Although athletes' physical confidence is challenged every day in their sport, an injury communicates to them that their body may no longer be capable of overcoming that challenge. The rehabilitation process is a daily reaffirmation of physical confidence in which injured athletes prove to themselves that their body will sustain them under physical stress. As healing occurs and function returns, physical confidence must increase until athletes believe that they can achieve a complete recovery and return to their previous level of performance. Physical confidence can also be increased by having injured athletes participate in a rigorous physical conditioning program apart from rehabilitation of the injured area (Steadman, 1982). This allows them to maintain and even surpass their preinjury level of general fitness, thereby bolstering their physical confidence regarding their injury and strengthening their belief in their overall readiness to return to sport when they have completed rehabilitation.

Athletes can further develop their physical confidence by acknowledging the progress they experience during rehabilitation. Direct successful experience is the most effective means to building confidence (Bandura, 1977). To that end, the rehabilitation staff should emphasize noticeable gains in range of motion, strength, and other relevant physical parameters. This recognition will give injured athletes renewed confidence that their body is again becoming capable of sustaining itself under the stresses that they place upon it.

Return-to-Sport Confidence

The final psychological hurdle for rehabilitating athletes is regaining their confidence that they can perform at or above their preinjury level. Injured athletes must believe that they are completely healed and that they have fully rehabilitated their injury. They need to have confidence that they were able to maintain their physical conditioning and their technical abilities during rehabilitation. Return-to-sport confidence is discussed in more detail in Chapter 11.

Rehabilitating the Confidence "Muscle"

Confidence can be thought of as a muscle that, like the physically injured area, also becomes injured. If the confidence "muscle" is not rehabilitated along with the damaged area, atrophy will occur and healing will not be complete. A still-injured confidence muscle will slow the rehabilitation process and make a full return to sport unlikely.

An injured confidence muscle that expresses itself as negative thinking, emotions, and physiology is a significant obstacle to recovery and return to sport. The injury causes athletes to doubt whether their body is capable of handling the demands placed on it. It also causes them to question whether they will be able to perform at a high level again. The injured confidence muscle also produces a negative attitude toward rehabilitation and return to sport. Giving injured athletes confidence-building "therapy" will help heal and condition the confidence muscle in preparation for return to sport.

Walk Strong

Humans are fundamentally physical beings. Thoughts and emotions are physical occurrences that are affected by other physical activity. Injured athletes can influence what they think and how they feel by the way they walk, move, and carry themselves.

The psychological and emotional burden of an injury is often expressed physically in terms of slow and labored gait and negative body language, which in turn exacerbate the negative thoughts and feelings caused by the injury. This is especially evident with lower extremity injuries that result in limping or use of crutches. Injured athletes can counter this negative impact by using their body to positively influence their thoughts and emotions. They can learn to "walk strong." This action produces positive physical changes in movement and body language, including walking with the chin up, the shoulders back, and an energetic step, as well as maintaining erect posture, resulting in positive thoughts and feelings. When injured athletes consistently walk strong, their thoughts and emotions become stronger and more positive too.

Talk Strong

When athletes are injured, it is common for them to talk negatively about their injury, for example, "My leg is never going to heal," or "I can't make it through rehab." This causes them to think negatively and feel bad. In contrast, when injured athletes talk positively, they think and feel more positively. The rehabilitation staff can bolster this aspect of confidence therapy by encouraging injured athletes to "talk strong," for example, "I am feeling better every day" or "I can't wait to start playing again."

Thought-Stopping

Thought-stopping involves increasing injured athletes' awareness of their negative thinking and talking and replacing the negativity with positive statements (Cautela & Wisocki, 1977). It helps the athletes to strengthen their confidence muscle. Thought-stopping involves several steps. First, injured athletes need to become aware of their negative thoughts. The rehabilitation staff facilitate this awareness by pointing out incidences when the athletes are negative. It is also useful for the athletes to note in writing whenever they think or say something negative. Second, injured athletes can use a trigger word such as *stop* or *positive* to interrupt the negativity (Bunker, Williams, & Zinsser, 1993). Finally, they can replace the negative thought with a positive statement.

MOTIVATION IN REHABILITATION

Motivation is the psychological issue that influences rehabilitation most directly (Brewer, 1994; Grove & Gordon, 1992; Pollard, 1994). For a rehabilitation program to be effective, patients must be motivated to stay with it. Any decline in motivation will result in a drop in adherence to the progam, which will in turn slow rehabilitation and hinder return to sport.

Rehabilitation motivation involves being able to fully adhere to the physical therapy regimen in the face of pain, fatigue, boredom, frustration, setbacks, and the desire to do other, less unpleasant activities. Motivation is so important to rehabilitation because it is one of the few aspects of injury management that is entirely within the control of the patient.

The importance of addressing motivation during rehabilitation has been noted by many sports medicine professionals and psychologists (Fisher, Mullins, & Frye, 1993; Grove & Gordon, 1992; Pollard, 1994). Athletic trainers have also indicated that motivation is a quality that separates athletes who cope well with an injury from those who do not (Wiese et al., 1991). Research has shown that motivation significantly influences physical therapy attendance and effort during rehabilitation sessions (Duda et al., 1989).

Motivation also plays a role in adherence to physical therapy regimens outside of the rehabilitation facility. Motivation affects all aspects of the injury management process, including physical conditioning, mental training, and lifestyle issues such as sleep, diet, daily stressors, and social support.

To ensure that injured athletes maintain their motivation, the rehabilitation staff should be alert to symptoms of low motivation. Common signs of reduced motivation include a decline in attendance at physical therapy sessions, not finishing required exercises and procedures, and poor focus, intensity, and effort during physical therapy. Indirect indications include unclear, easily achievable, or unreachable goals; using unfounded pain as a way of getting out of physical therapy; and having regular and unexplainable excuses for missing physical therapy.

The ongoing presence of any of these warning signs should indicate to the rehabilitation staff that a discussion with the athlete about the importance of motivation is warranted. A dialogue conducted in a cooperative, problem-solving tone can lead to solutions to some of these motivational barriers. What is most important is that patients appreciate the impact that motivation has on rehabilitation, recognize their level of motivation, and take active steps to maximize their motivation throughout the course of their recovery.

DEVELOPING AND MAINTAINING MOTIVATION

Loss of motivation at some point during rehabilitation is normal and expected, even for the most determined athletes. Motivation often declines during periods of pain and at the midpoint of rehabilitation, when injured athletes grow weary of the rehabilitation process yet are still a long way from completing rehabilitation. Because of the essential role that motivation plays in the rehabilitation phase of the injury management process, injured athletes need to be shown tools that they can use to maintain their motivation.

Focus on Long-Term Goals

It is easy for rehabilitating athletes to get so caught up in the pain and frustration of physical therapy sessions that they lose sight of why they are enduring such discomfort, resulting in a drop in motivation. To counter this unproductive focus, the rehabilitation staff should remind athletes of why they are tolerating the pain and tedium of physical therapy, namely, their determination to heal as fast as possible and return to their sport as soon as possible. One way to redirect their focus toward the future is to have them write down and read their long-term goals for their sport every day. Having them state their long-term goals and then imagine what they want to accomplish can bolster motivation during difficult periods. Another method is to have athletes identify their greatest competitor and place that competitor's name or photo where they can see it as a constant reminder of what they need to do to get back to competing against that person.

Variety in Rehabilitation

One of most difficult aspects of rehabilitation is the repetitiousness involved in physical therapy, which can breed boredom and complacency and cause loss of motivation, effort, intensity, and focus. To counter this motivation-draining influence, variety should be incorporated into rehabilitation sessions. Like cross-training in physical conditioning programs, performing different exercises to rehabilitate an injury will keep physical therapy novel, stimulating, and interesting. Doing new exercises will require injured athletes to focus more and apply themselves more purposefully and intensely in their physical therapy sessions.

Rehab Partner

Rehabilitation is difficult to do alone. There is just too much pain and discomfort for injured athletes to give their best effort all of the time. It is often the responsibility of the rehabilitation staff to push patients when their motivation lags. The staff cannot always be there to provide that extrinsic motivation, however, and they also do not want patients to become dependent on them. So, a useful strategy is to identify rehab partners who can work together and motivate each other to give their best effort.

There are many days during the course of rehabilitation when an athlete just does not feel like going to physical therapy. With rehab partners, however, chances are one of them will be motivated. Also, with rehab partners there is a sense of commitment and responsibility not only to self but also to someone else. So, if a rehab partner does not show up for physical therapy, that partner is not letting down just self but is also disappointing someone else. In choosing rehab partners, the stage of rehabilitation and the ability to match physical therapy schedules should be considered. Most important, however, the two injured athletes must get along well and be willing to push each other to attain their recovery goals.

STRESS IN REHABILITATION

Stress may be the most prevalent and debilitating influence on rehabilitation. Stress is considered to be a negative psychological and physical response to a perceived threat (Hackfort & Schwenkmezger, 1993). Stress occurs in injured athletes when they view their injury and the subsequent rehabilitation as a threat to their physical health and sense of self-worth. Brewer, Petitpas, Van Raalte, Sklar, and Ditmar (1995) found that a third of injured athletes displayed behavioral indications of stress. Additionally, Brewer, Van Raalte, and Linder (1991) reported that stress was among the most frequently seen psychological reactions to injury.

Effects of Stress on Rehabilitation

Stress interferes with rehabilitation at several essential levels. Initially, it hurts key psychological contributors to rehabilitation, including confidence, motivation, and focus (Meichenbaum, 1985; Nideffer, 1989; Schonfeld, 1992). Stress reduces injured athletes' confidence by causing them to doubt aspects of their rehabilitation program. Stress also inhibits their motivation to adhere to their physical therapy regimen. Stress can also cause athletes to focus on debilitating aspects of the injury rather than on efforts to facilitate recovery.

The physical price of stress includes greater perceptions of pain (Lee, 1993), increased need for pain medication (Asmundson & Norton, 1995), and reduced healing (Holden-Lund, 1988). Stress inhibits breathing and the intake of oxygen (Hackfort & Schwenkmezger, 1993; Harris & Williams, 1993), causing muscle tension, restricting blood flow (Navateur, 1992), and increasing pain (Lee, 1993). Stress also disrupts sleep (Giesecke, 1987) and appetite (Miles, 1985) and has the cumulative effect of slowing healing by decreasing the efficiency of the immune system (Eysenck, 1994; Fredrikson, Furst, Ekander, & Rotstein, 1993).

Symptoms of Stress in Rehabilitation

The most harmful thing about stress is its pervasive impact on rehabilitation. Stress negatively affects injured athletes physically, cognitively, emotionally, and socially and also diminishes rehabilitation performance. Understanding the symptoms of stress (see Table 8.2) helps to identify their presence through observation or questioning of the patient. Following is a summary of the symptoms:

- *Physical.* Physical symptoms of stress include muscle tension and bracing, short and rapid breathing, decreased coordination and balance, and fatigue (Heil, 1993). General physical indications are minor muscle pulls and strain, nagging illness, recurrent physical complaints, and sleeping problems.
- *Cognitive.* Common cognitive signs involve excessive negativity, overcritical self-evaluations, statements of low confidence about various aspects of rehabilitation, extreme thinking, and unrealistic expectations. Another interesting and subtle cognitive symptom is an overnarrowing of focus (Andersen & Williams, 1989; Weltman & Egstrom, 1966), which may show itself in inattentiveness to instructions, forgetfulness, or poor form in physical therapy exercises.
- *Emotional.* Stress is most powerfully expressed emotionally. These emotional expressions are almost always negative and can be used as a barometer of the severity of the stress. As a general rule, the stronger the emotions, the more stress the patient is feeling. Typical emotional symptoms of stress are anger, depression, irritability, moodiness, and impatience with rehabilitation (Heil, 1993). In general, emotions that seem inappropriate, out of place, or excessively strong are clear indicators of stress.
- *Social.* The social impact of stress is significant because it removes one of the most important buffers to stress, namely, social support. Injured athletes tend to communicate less, withdraw socially, and show intolerance and abruptness

TABLE 8.2

Symptoms of Stress in Rehabilitation

Physical	Muscle tension and bracing
	Short, choppy breathing
	Decreased coordination
	Fatigue
	Rushed speech
	Fast pace in physical therapy
	Minor secondary injuries
	Nagging illness
	Recurrent physical complaints
	Sleeping problems
Cognitive	Excessive negativity
	Too self-critical
	Statements of low confidence in rehabilitation
	Extreme thinking
	Unrealistic expectations
	Overnarrowing of focus
Emotional	Anger
	Depression
	Irritability
	Moodiness
	Impatience
Social	Less communicative
	Social withdrawal
	Intolerance of others
	Abruptness with others
Performance	Overall decline in motivation and enjoyment in rehabilitation
	Loss of interest in sport and other activities
	Nervousness and physical tension in physical therapy
	Trying too hard in physical therapy
	"Give up" syndrome in response to obstacles and setbacks
	Decrease in school or work performance

Note. Adapted from *Psychological Approaches to Sports Injury Rehabilitation* (p. 149), by J. Taylor and S. Taylor, 1997, Austin, TX: PRO-ED. Copyright 1997 by PRO-ED, Inc. Reprinted with permission.

toward others. This reaction can cause them to become more isolated from those they need most—the rehabilitation staff, teammates, family, and friends.

- *Performance*. Stress influences rehabilitation performance by hurting motivation and interest in physical therapy, producing tight performance in physical therapy exercises and the appearance that the athletes are trying too hard. At the same time, their tolerance to pain, frustration, and boredom is low, so they tend to give up when faced with minor obstacles or setbacks. It is also common to see this "give up" response generalize to other areas of their lives, such as school or work, where a decline in grades or productivity is seen.

Causes and Prevention of Stress in Rehabilitation

All injured athletes experience some debilitating stress at some point during their rehabilitation. Stress is caused by a variety of physical, psychological, and social factors (see Table 8.3). Although a direct response to indications of stress is important, the best way to deal with stress is to prevent it. By addressing the causes proactively, many of the reactions that injured athletes experience can be prevented. A nice benefit of prevention is that some basic strategies can be incorporated directly into the structure of rehabilitation programs, daily activities, and daily physical therapy sessions (see Table 8.3).

Physical

The main physical cause of stress is the pervasive pain that injured athletes experience throughout rehabilitation. A well-managed medication program for pain control can alleviate much of the physical stress by reducing the pain that causes it. In addition, use of nonpharmacological pain management (see Chapter 9) can provide further benefit to injured athletes, not only by reducing pain but also by decreasing the need for medication and enhancing the athletes' sense of control over their stress. Strategies to reduce the stress that increases pain are discussed later in this chapter.

Stress is also caused by the considerable demands that rehabilitation and healing put on the body. Especially with serious injuries that involve lengthy recovery, the ongoing and unrelenting strain of rehabilitation can lead to stress reactions. The energy necessary for rehabilitation and healing also places great stress on the body. Injured athletes rarely appreciate these demands and attempt to maintain their usual active lifestyles.

Table 8.3

Causes and Prevention of Stress in Rehabilitation

	Causes	Prevention
Physical	Pain	Pain management
	Rehabilitation	Continue noninjury development in sport
	Healing	Mental training for return to sport and concern for reinjury
	Falling behind in athletic development	Complementary practices: yoga, therapeutic massage, tai chi
	Returning to form	
	Reinjury	
Psychological	Low confidence	Rehabilitation education
	Threat to self-esteem	Build and maintain confidence
	Catastrophizing	Establish realistic goals and expectations
	Lack of familiarity, predictability, control	Develop rehabilitation routines
	Unrealistic expectations	Complementary practices: transcendental meditation, relaxation response
Social	Pressure from others	Create diverse social support network
	Loss of social reinforcement	Educate social support network about rehabilitation
		Communicate openly with individuals in social network
		Explore other rewarding activities

Note. From *Psychological Approaches to Sports Injury Rehabilitation* (pp. 151–152), by J. Taylor and S. Taylor, 1997, Austin, TX: PRO-ED. Copyright 1997 by PRO-ED, Inc. Reprinted with permission.

Education about the impact of rehabilition and suggestions about how to moderate their activities within the physical demands of rehabilitation and healing help athletes to manage the demands and reduce the related stress.

Psychological

Injured athletes need to understand that stress is a normal and anticipated reaction to injury and rehabilitation. However, stress is a problem when it becomes an ever-present and debilitating response to injury. Low confidence is a primary source of stress among injured athletes. If they have doubts about whether they can recover fully, they will feel overwhelmed and incapable of handling the demands that will be placed upon them in rehabilitation. This uncertainty, in turn, will produce stress. A natural reaction to these doubts is the emergence of "catastrophizing," or extreme thinking (J.Taylor & Taylor, 1997). These irrational thoughts (e.g., "I will never recover," or "I will be crippled for life") further harm confidence and increase stress. The best way to build confidence is with the techniques discussed earlier in this chapter under "Rehabilitating the Confidence 'Muscle.'"

One of the most difficult aspects of athletes' injury rehabilitation is their lack of familiarity with the process and lack of control over it. Injured athletes simply do not know enough about the injury management process to have some sense that they can master it. This lack of understanding results in feelings of helplessness and stress. Information offers injured athletes familiarity, predictability, and control in all phases of rehabilitation. This process involves educating injured athletes about all relevant aspects of their injury and rehabilitation.

As injured athletes near the end of their rehabilitation, they have a tendency to assume that the stressful part of the injury management process is behind them. In reality, however, the transition to return to sport can produce another completely different stress response. As return to sport nears, injured athletes' attention turns to questions about whether rehabilitation has been successful and whether they can perform at a high level again. They may also feel stress about the potential for reinjury. These concerns are discussed further in Chapter 11.

Social

A variety of social issues can cause stress in injured athletes. Competitive athletes often feel pressure from coaches, teammates, family, friends, and media to return to sport sooner than is prudent. These pressures may be due to a team's need to win, financial demands, or overinvolvement of family, friends, community, or media. This social pressure can cause stress because it is both uncontrollable by the athlete and, at the same time, highly invasive and unavoidable.

Educating individuals in the injured athlete's social network—family, friends, coaches, and so on—about the positive and negative impact they can have on the athlete can lead to their helping rather than hurting the athlete. Helping these individuals gain an appreciation of the rehabilitation process can give them realistic expectations about the athlete's recovery and help them put their own needs in perspective, so that they will not put undue and harmful pressure on the athlete to return to sport sooner than is advisable. As part of this education process, the injured athlete should be encouraged to talk to family, friends, coaches, teammates, and others to foster an empathetic view of what the athlete is going through and to enhance the social support that the athlete is given.

A difficult aspect of injury and rehabilitation is that injured athletes are removed from parts of their lives that are fulfilling and supportive. Not only are they forced to deal with an injury, but they must also do it in the absence of people who give them a great deal of support. These potential causes of stress can be prevented by having the athletes take active steps to stay connected with their primary sources of social support and to stay involved in their sport as much as is feasible.

Mastering Stress in Rehabilitation

Although attempts to prevent stress are important and valuable, stress is an inevitable part of the rehabilitation experience. Because of this, it is useful to offer injured athletes some simple and practical strategies that they can use to relieve the stress that they will experience and limit any negative effects it might have on their rehabilitation. Having the tools to master their stress during rehabilitation has several benefits. It offers psychological advantages such as a greater sense of control, enhanced confidence, a higher level of relaxation, and a more positive focus. It also provides physical benefits, such as less pain, fewer uncomfortable physical symptoms, and improved healing.

Breathing

The foremost physical reaction of humans to stress is to hold their breath. As discussed earlier, this inhibits oxygen intake, causes muscle tension, and slows healing (Harris & Williams, 1993). The simplest way to relieve stress is to take slow, deep breaths. Deep breathing gets adequate oxygen to the muscles, eases muscle tension, gives injured athletes a greater sense of control over their body, and redirects focus away from negative aspects of the injury such as pain.

Part of the value of breathing is increasing injured athletes' awareness of their breathing during physical therapy. Often, they hold their breath or take short, abrupt breaths. Showing them how to breathe properly during rehabilitation exercises will not only reduce immediate stress but also be beneficial upon their return to sport.

Many breathing techniques have become popularized, including diaphragmatic, rhythmic, and concentrated breathing (Harris & Williams, 1993). However, we advocate a simple deep-breathing technique that involves a slow and deep inhale, a brief hold when the lungs are full, and a slow and long exhale. Deep breathing can be incorporated directly into physical therapy sessions. Before beginning an exercise, injured athletes can take two deep breaths. During the exercise, they can breathe out on exertion. After the effort of the exercise, injured athletes can take two more deep breaths to relax the body.

Relaxation Training

The most harmful reaction to stress is the excessive muscle tension and bracing that results from the body's attempt to protect itself (Heil, 1993). Muscle tension increases pain, inhibits blood flow, and restricts range of motion. The two primary benefits of relaxation training are to enhance injured athletes' awareness of their muscles and to increase their control over muscle tension (Harris & Williams, 1993). Injured athletes learn to recognize muscle tension when they experience it and actively relax their muscles should they feel tension.

Two kinds of relaxation training have been found to be effective and practical for injured athletes: passive relaxation (J. Taylor, 2001) and progressive relaxation (Jacobson, 1938). Passive relaxation involves deep breathing and allowing tension to drain from their body, inducing a state of muscle relaxation. It is most useful for injured athletes who experience low to moderate muscle tension and who want to feel more relaxed and comfortable. Progressive relaxation combines tensing and relaxing muscles and deep breathing. It is most effective for injured athletes who are not aware of their muscular states and who have substantial muscle tension in response to stress. Relaxation training is most beneficial when it is incorporated into rehabilitation, specifically, at the end of physical therapy sessions when pain is usually significant. Both types of relaxation are most effective when done lying comfortably in a quiet place.

Music

Music is also an excellent tool for reducing stress because it has the ability to alter many facets of human functioning, including attitude, mood, emotions, and physiology. Music can enhance rehabilitation by inducing states of relaxation, reducing stress, and generating positive emotions. Music is also a useful accompaniment to relaxation training.

Therapeutic Massage

Therapeutic massage is highly effective at reducing stress because it acts directly on the muscular effects of stress. Typical responses to therapeutic massage include release of muscle tension, induction of a general state of physical comfort, and improved blood flow to the injured area (Ferrell-Torry & Glick, 1993; Goats, 1994). Therapeutic massage also reduces swelling, encourages healing, and allows the body to recuperate from the demands of rehabilitation (Kaard & Tostinbo, 1989; Zanolla, Monzeglio, & Balzarini, 1984).

INTENSITY AND REHABILITATION

Intensity is one of the most important concepts in sports performance (J. Taylor, 2001). Athletes understand that they need intensity to perform their best in training and competition. They also realize that intensity must vary depending on the sport or aspect of the sport in which they participate. If athletes recognize the value of rehabilitation as athletic performance, they will also value the importance of intensity in their rehabilitation efforts. Intensity can assist injured athletes in maximizing the value of their physical therapy sessions and in keeping their psychological skills sharp while away from their sport. Focusing on intensity during rehabilitation shows injured athletes how different degrees of intensity are needed for different physical therapy exercises, how intensity affects their physical performance, and how regulating intensity can enhance the quality of their physical therapy efforts and benefit them when they return to sport.

Learning About Intensity

Using intensity effectively in rehabilitation starts with understanding what levels of intensity go best with different physical therapy procedures. Injured athletes can determine whether it is better to be relaxed, moderate, or intense for various physical therapy exercises such as resistance training (high), agility (moderate), and stretching (low). They can then monitor their own intensity before physical therapy exercises to see whether it is at a level appropriate for the particular exercise. They can also experiment with their level of intensity during physical therapy to see what effect it has on their efforts. For example, if they raise their intensity, what happens to their flexibility? Or, if they become very relaxed, what effect does it have on their strength? Using this method, injured athletes can learn what level of intensity works best for different facets of rehabilitation. They can also transfer this knowledge of intensity to their sport to better understand how it affects their sport training and competitive performances.

Intensity Regulation

Once injured athletes understand the ideal intensity for various physical therapy procedures, they can check their intensity and adjust it before every exercise by using "psych-down" or "psych-up" techniques. Psych-down techniques were discussed earlier in this chapter under "Mastering Stress in Rehabilitation." These methods, which include deep breathing, passive and progressive relaxation, and listening to music, can all be used to reduce intensity. Psych-down techniques are most appropriate for rehabilitation exercises relevant to range of motion, muscular stretching, and coordination.

Psych-up techniques aim at raising intensity for increased energy and power. Psych-up techniques are best used for physical therapy exercises that train strength and quickness in short bursts. Elevating intensity involves raising heart rate, respiration, blood flow, and adrenaline to bolster effort and explosiveness. At a basic level, injured athletes can "rev their engines," which entails directly increasing their physiological activity with walking, running, riding a stationary bike, or other movement that stimulates their sympathetic nervous system. Injured athletes can also use breathing that is consistent with the ensuing exercise. For example, before stretching they can take slow, deep breaths, and before weight lifting, they can take short, hard breaths. High-energy body language, including clenching a fist or slapping a thigh, can also be used to increase intensity. Psychological strategies to raise intensity include stopping negative thoughts (e.g., "I can't take this anymore," or "I'm never going to recover") and using high-energy self-talk (e.g., "Come on!" or "Stay with it!").

FOCUS IN REHABILITATION

Focus is the most underappreciated psychological contributor to rehabilitation. Because it is so misunderstood, most people are unaware of the impact it has on other psychological factors and on the quality of physical therapy and the overall rehabilitation process. The scant research on focus in rehabilitation has indicated that focusing on short-term goals can facilitate athletes' coping with injury (Wiese et al., 1991) and that appropriate focus is a criterion for athletes' effective return to sport (Pollard, 1994). Nideffer (1983) found that an injury tends to increase physiological stress and produces preoccupation with the injured area, an example of poor focus, which degrades the quality of physical therapy.

What Is Focus?

The attentional field is everything outside of people (e.g., sights and sounds) and everything inside of people (e.g., thoughts, emotions, physical responses) on which they could focus at any one time (Nideffer, 1976). Focus is the ability to attend to various internal and external cues in the attentional field and to be able to shift focus to other cues as the need arises.

Injured athletes have a wide range of facilitating and interfering cues in their attentional field on which they could focus during the course of rehabilitation. Poor focus involves injured athletes' attending to internal and external cues that interfere with their physical therapy. Internal interfering cues include negative thoughts, stress, and preoccupation with the injured area. External interfering cues consist of pressure from others to recover quickly, distractions during physical therapy, and worries about falling behind other competitors. This poor focus lowers motivation, hurts confidence, increases stress, and reduces the quality of physical therapy sessions.

Ideal focus involves focusing only on internal and external cues that will help rehabilitation. Internal facilitating cues consist of pain (as information), confidence, tension, and proprioceptive responses. External facilitating cues include exercise instruction, encouragement from others, and feedback from rehabilitation equipment. The ability to effectively focus on facilitating cues at the appropriate time and to be able to shift focus to other facilitating cues at other times is essential to quality rehabilitation.

Long-Term Versus Short-Term Focus

Having both a short-term and a long-term focus can be useful to injured athletes at different points in their recovery. Particularly for athletes who have a protracted rehabilitation ahead of them, having a long-term focus can be intimidating and foreboding. To these athletes, a complete recovery may seem to be so far off as to be unreachable. These athletes may need to see recovery as a day-to-day process in which they focus solely on their most immediate needs in rehabilitation. With this short-term focus, they can concentrate on specific components of physical therapy that they can handle and over which they feel some sense of control.

A long-term focus can also provide injured athletes with some benefits. There are times when the everyday minutiae of physical therapy are overwhelming. Injured athletes feel pain, stress, and frustration. They may say things like, "I'm never going to get through this," or "I can't take it anymore." This is the time when a long-term focus can draw their attention away from the drudgery and tedium of the present and redirect it onto the reason for their going through such discomfort. This long-term perspective enables them to focus on more positive and motivating aspects of recovery.

CHAPTER 9

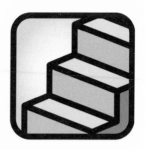

Facilitating Rehabilitation

In addition to the mental stratagems for enhancing the quality of rehabilitation described in Chapter 8, several other strategies can be used to facilitate the recovery process. These approaches are devoted to positively influencing essential physical, psychological, and social issues that directly affect the effectiveness of rehabilitation. These strategies are not well known among injured athletes or commonly addressed in a formal way during rehabilitation. Yet, there is strong research support for their value in encouraging recovery. Answers to the following questions can provide injured athletes with additional means to maximize the rehabilitation process:

- What can I do to counteract the physical toll that rehabilitation will take on me?

- What can I do to keep my use of pain medication to a minimum?

- How can rehabilitation imagery facilitate my recovery?

- What role do other people play in the quality of my rehabilitation?

- I've heard of athletes who made amazing recoveries from injuries like mine. What did they do to have such fast recoveries?

The answers to these five questions can provide injured athletes with special information and techniques that are not often considered in the traditional injury management process. Yet, this knowledge can give the athletes physical and psychological benefits that can significantly improve the quality of rehabilitation and speed return to sport.

IMPORTANCE OF REST
IN REHABILITATION

Unless athletes have been injured before, they are not usually aware of the physical toll that rehabilitation takes on them. The healing, the energy put into physical therapy, the pain that accompanies recovery, and the general disruption of life can all weigh heavily on injured athletes as they progress through rehabilitation. A common mistake many injured athletes make is to try to maintain their normal lifestyle of work, school, social events, and other activities while engaging in a rigorous physical therapy program. Injured athletes usually do not fully appreciate that healing requires considerable physical energy as the body works to mend the injured area. Patients often complain of being very tired even though they seem to be doing less than normal.

Healing can be bolstered by ensuring that all available energy is directed toward mending the injured area. Physical therapy is also physically demanding and draining. Injured athletes do not always appreciate that rehabilitation is a form of physical conditioning that focuses on a specific area. In addition, it is physical effort directed toward an area that is not accustomed to such intense demands. The stresses of physical therapy are further exacerbated by the pain, which depletes energy, slows healing, and hinders the rehabilitation process (Heil, 1993). It is essential that injured athletes understand the significant stress that the injury, healing, and physical therapy place on the body and what they can do to ensure that their body has the capacity to maximize their rehabilitation (see Table 9.1)—especially the critical role of rest.

Rest is an integral part of the rehabilitation process. It can guard against the damaging effects of the physical and psychological demands of rehabilitation. Injured athletes must be convinced of the value of rest as an essential part of healing and recovery (Israel, 1976; Kindermann, 1988). Injured athletes often do not realize that it is during rest, not during exercise, that healing occurs and gains are made. Rest also protects injured athletes from the normal stresses of daily life and the general grind of the recovery process.

TABLE 9.1
Patient Education Guide: Importance of Rest

1. Rehabilitation places significant demands on the body
   a. Pain saps energy
   b. Healing takes energy
   c. Physical therapy requires effort
   d. Injured athletes cannot maintain the same active lifestyle as when they were not injured
2. Warning signs of fatigue
   a. Ongoing tiredness
   b. Sleeping difficulties
   c. Sore muscles
   d. Slow recovery from previous day's physical therapy
   e. Minor secondary injuries
   f. Lingering illness (indicates that immune system is overloaded)
   g. Loss of motivation
   h. Depressed mood
3. Adjust lifestyle
   a. Reduce intensity of lifestyle (e.g., workload or school load, social activities, general physical conditioning program)
   b. Adjust nutritional needs
   c. Use therapeutic massage
   d. Earlier bedtimes
   e. Take naps as needed
4. Incorporate rest in rehabilitation
   a. Establish mandatory rest day
   b. Periodize weekly physical therapy regimen
   c. Make rehabilitation program flexible based on how injured athlete feels each day
   d. Listen to the body

Incorporating Rest into Rehabilitation

Injured athletes should understand that everything they do, whether work or play, expends energy that could slow healing and recovery. With this understanding, they can modify their daily activities to ensure that they devote sufficient energy to their rehabilitation efforts. Common modifications include less intensive school or work schedules, less socializing, and a reduced noninjury exercise regimen. Injured athletes can also adjust their nutrition needs. This may involve reducing intake, because they are not training as hard as they were before the injury, or eating more to meet the added physical demands of rehabilitation. A therapeutic massage is another proactive step that injured athletes can take to bolster recuperation. Injured athletes should also avail themselves of opportunities for additional sleep. Going to bed earlier and taking afternoon naps are two common ways to ensure that they are giving their body every chance to gain rest.

To convey the importance of rest in rehabilitation, the rehabilitation staff should emphasize it within the context of physical therapy. This can be accomplished in two ways. A mandatory rest day should be scheduled into the weekly physical therapy regimen. Also, physical therapy can be arranged with alternating days of high- and low-intensity rehabilitation and can be flexible enough to adjust to how injured athletes feel on any given day.

Warning Signs of Fatigue

Fatigue can be a significant barrier to recovery. It inhibits healing (Kindermann, 1988; Tharp & Barnes, 1989) and increases the risk of healing cycles (see Chapter 6) and reinjury. It can also lower motivation, reduce adherence to the physical therapy program, and decrease effort and intensity in rehabilitation exercises. Indications of fatigue include ongoing tiredness, difficulty sleeping, sore muscles, poor recovery, minor secondary injuries, lingering illness (Kuipers & Keizer, 1988), depressed mood, loss of enthusiasm, and poor-quality rehabilitation.

An essential lesson injured athletes must learn is to listen to and respond to how their body is feeling. The body will tell them when they are becoming fatigued. What is necessary, however, is that they recognize the warning signs and take steps to reverse the impending exhaustion by actively seeking out its various forms.

PAIN MANAGEMENT

Pain is the greatest barrier to effective rehabilitation. Yet, it is rare for rehabilitation professionals to educate injured athletes as to how pain affects them and how they can manage it without medication. One study of athletic trainers indicated that they did not view pain management techniques as tools that can aid in rehabilitation or improve the quality of their work with injured athletes (Larson, Starkey, & Zaichkowsky, 1996; Wiese, Weiss, & Yukelson, 1991). This finding may suggest a lack of knowledge of nonanalgesic pain management or insufficient time to implement such strategies (Larson et al., 1996), because extensive research has indicated that pain management techniques are effective in reducing pain without pharmacological intervention (Berntzen, 1987).

Injured athletes can gain several benefits from using nonanalgesic pain management. Physically, they will experience less pain and will be able to avoid unnecessary medication. Psychologically, their sense of control will increase, and they will feel less stressed and more confident. However, nonpharmacological pain management is not an absolute replacement for medication but rather a useful complement to traditional pain management. Injured athletes should consult with their physician in determining the best means of pain management.

Pain management strategies can be classified as either pain reduction or pain focusing (see Figure 9.1). The goal of pain reduction is to lessen autonomic activity that increases pain, for example, peripheral vasoconstriction, muscle spasm, and muscular bracing (Cousins & Phillips, 1985). Pain reduction occurs by inducing physiological relaxation and the related decrease in parasympathetic nervous system activity, thus reducing the actual pain that is felt. Pain reduction techniques include deep breathing, muscle relaxation training, and therapeutic massage, discussed in Chapter 8.

Pain focusing consists of directing attention to or away from the pain to decrease the perception of pain. Pain focusing has been broadly classified into dissociative and associative strategies (Morgan & Pollock, 1977). Dissociative focusing involves directing attention away from the pain that the patient is experiencing. The rationale is that if patients are not paying attention to their pain, they will perceive the pain as less intense (Wack & Turk, 1984). Associative focusing entails directing attention to the pain and interpreting it in a different way to change its perception and meaning.

Six types of pain-focusing techniques have been shown to be effective in reducing the perception of pain (Fernandez & Turk, 1986). *External focus* involves directing attention externally to either emotionally (e.g., music, film, television, literature) or intellectually (e.g., playing chess, constructing a model airplane, engaging in conversation) absorbing activities. *Pleasant imagining* involves generating pleasurable images such as lying on a beach or floating in space. *Neutral imagining* entails imagining an intellectually absorbing activity such as playing chess or building a house. *Rhythmic cognitive activity* involves focusing on a repetitious or structured task such as counting, meditating, or singing. In *pain acknowledgment,*

Pain Reduction

> Deep breathing—emphasis on slow, deep, rhythmic breathing

> Muscle relaxation—passive or progressive relaxation

> Meditation—repetitive focusing on mantra or breathing

> Therapeutic massage—manual manipulation of muscles, tendons, and ligaments

Pain Focus

> External focus—listening to relaxing or inspiring music; watching a movie; playing chess

> Soothing imagery—generating calming images, such as lying on a beach, floating in space

> Neutral imaginings—imagining playing chess or constructing a model airplane

> Rhythmic cognitive activity—saying the alphabet backward; meditation

> Pain acknowledgment—giving pain a "hot" color, such as red, then changing it to a less painful "cool" color, such as blue

> Dramatic coping—seeing pain as part of an epic challenge to overcome insurmountable odds

> Situational assessment—evaluating the causes of pain to take steps to reduce it

---

Figure 9.1. Pain management techniques. *Note.* From *Psychological Approaches to Sports Injury Rehabilitation* (p. 142), by J. Taylor and S. Taylor, 1997, Austin, TX: PRO-ED. Copyright 1997 by PRO-ED, Inc. Reprinted with permission.

patients use imagery to endow the pain with physical qualities such as size, color, and texture as a means of making the pain more tangible and more controllable. *Dramatic coping* involves viewing the pain in the context of a great challenge or an epic journey.

REHABILITATION IMAGERY

Mental imagery shows tremendous promise in supporting a diverse array of psychological and physical contributors to recovery. It is widely used in the sports world to enhance many aspects of athletic performance (Vealey & Walter, 1993), but only more recently has it been thought to be of value in bolstering the rehabilitation process (Green, 1992).

Research outside of sports medicine has reported the positive impact of mental imagery on immune system activity (Achterberg, 1991; Post-White, 1991), cancer (Achterberg, Mathews-Simonton, & Simonton, 1977; Fiore, 1988), psoriasis (Gaston, Crombez, & Dupuis, 1989), and ulcers, fractures, and hip disarticulations (Korn, 1983). It has also documented the ability of mental imagery to alter physiological activity such as muscle activity (Sheikh & Jordan, 1983), vasoconstriction (Sarno, 1984), blood-glucose levels, and skin temperature (Barber, 1978). Within sports medicine, rehabilitation imagery has been strongly advocated (e.g., Arnheim, 1989; Rotella & Heyman, 1993), and it has also been associated with more timely rehabilitation. Yet, results from a study of athletic trainers indicate that they did not believe that mental imagery was a useful strategy for enhancing injured athletes' coping with rehabilitation (Wiese et al., 1991).

Types of Rehabilitation Imagery

Three types of imagery—healing, soothing, and performance—are useful in the healing, rehabilitation, and return to sport of injured athletes. These forms of rehabilitation imagery can encourage physical, mental, and athletic development during recovery and return to sport.

- *Healing imagery.* Healing imagery involves having injured athletes imagine the damaged area mending and healing. Injured athletes need to have a clear picture of the injured area and what it looks like when healed. This can be done with illustrations and X rays of the injured area. Over the period of rehabilitation, healing imagery may physiologically facilitate the healing process. Just as important, it will build confidence and trust that the injured area is healing fully.
- *Soothing imagery.* Soothing imagery can be a useful technique for lessening pain (Fernandez & Turk, 1986). Injured athletes can see and feel themselves in a calm and peaceful place, for example, floating on a cloud. Soothing imagery reduces sympathetic nervous system activity, muscle tension, and other symptoms of stress (Heil, 1993). It has a dissociative effect of taking injured athletes' focus away from their pain and directing it toward more enjoyable images and feelings (Morgan & Pollock, 1977). The soothing images can foster positive emotions, which also ease pain.
- *Performance imagery.* Performance imagery is very important during rehabilitation because it counters the belief held by injured athletes that their athletic development is being halted and they are falling behind their competition. Performance imagery is a means for injured athletes to continue their progress in

the areas of technique, tactics, mental preparation, and competitive performance while they are recovering from injury. A program of regular performance imagery sessions in which injured athletes see and feel themselves performing in their sport can help reduce the "psychological atrophy" that can occur while they are away from their sport (Grove & Gordon, 1992; Rotella & Heyman, 1993; Weiss & Troxel, 1986).

Maximizing Rehabilitation Imagery

Effective rehabilitation imagery involves complete reproduction of the actual scenes. Imagery should include visual, auditory, kinesthetic, thought, and emotional aspects of the real experience. Rehabilitation imagery is more than just mental rehearsal. It is reexperiencing the actual scenes and performances that are imagined.

Like any skill, the quality of rehabilitation imagery improves with time and practice (D. Smith, 1987). Several key factors influence the value of rehabilitation imagery. By paying attention to these factors, injured athletes can maximize the benefit of all three types of rehabilitation imagery during the recovery process.

- *Imagery perspective.* Injured athletes can use one of two types of perspective—internal or external—when they engage in rehabilitation imagery (D. Smith, 1987). Internal perspective consists of seeing the imagined elements through their own eyes, just like they were actually there. For example, a sprinter sees herself running from inside her body with the finish line at the end of the lane ahead and sees her competitors out of the corners of her eyes. External perspective involves viewing the scene from outside their body, as if they were watching the scene on video. Both perspectives have proven to be equally effective in enhancing rehabilitation and athletic performance.
- *Imagery vividness.* Injured athletes often say that their imagery is blurry and unclear. Unclear imagery may be caused by lack of experience in using imagery or by athletes' unfamiliarity with the images they are trying to generate. Vivid images are realistic, detailed, and clear and include all of the requisite senses, thoughts, and emotions (D. Smith, 1987). Imagery is a skill that improves with practice.

Imagery vividness can be improved in several ways. To enhance healing imagery, injured athletes can learn more about the nature of the injury and concentrate on seeing it healing and becoming completely mended. For performance imagery, they can watch videos of themselves to get a better image of what they look like when they perform.

• *Imagery control.* For rehabilitation imagery to be effective, injured athletes must generate positive images, feelings, and performances. Yet, a commonly reported complaint is that, despite their best efforts, they cannot control their images and end up imagining negative images, feelings, and performances. Unfortunately, if injured athletes continually generate negative imagery, they will internalize the negative images (Tversky & Kahneman, 1973; Woolfolk, Parrish, & Murphy, 1985), and it will hurt confidence (Clark, 1960) and focus (Gregory, Cialdini, & Carpenter, 1982). Poor imagery control is usually due to lack of experience and practice with imagery; also, spontaneous replay of the injury may still be occurring.

When injured athletes experience poor imagery control, they should immediately correct it with positive imagery. Rehabilitation imagery can be thought of as a video inside the head. When athletes lose imagery control, they should rewind the video and "edit" it with positive images. Because imagery control is a skill, as the athletes become more experienced, positive images will become easier to generate.

• *Relaxation and imagery.* Rehabilitation imagery can be improved by combining it with relaxation exercises. Doing imagery while relaxed seems to enhance vividness and control (Greenspan & Feltz, 1989; Hellstedt, 1987), improve focus and imagery quality (Lang, 1977), and allow injured athletes to be more susceptible to positive imagery experiences (Taylor, Horevitz, & Balague, 1993).

Developing a Rehabilitation Imagery Program

Rehabilitation imagery is a universal technique for fostering physical, psychological, and emotional contributors to recovery. Like physical therapy, however, it is only useful if injured athletes use it on a consistent basis. To gain the greatest benefit, they should develop an organized rehabilitation imagery program that identifies what they want to focus on, establishes goals toward which to strive, and creates a schedule of rehabilitation imagery sessions.

• *Focus of the rehabilitation imagery.* Injured athletes can specify the type of healing, soothing, and performance imagery on which they want to focus. For each kind of imagery, they should indicate the particular area that they need to work on. For example, healing imagery might emphasize seeing and feeling a broken bone fusing back together and healing. Soothing imagery might focus on improving breathing and reducing muscle tension. Performance imagery might stress gaining a better understanding of tactics.

• *Goals of rehabilitation imagery.* Injured athletes should set goals for each area they plan to work on. These goals should specify the area to be worked on, how often this type of imagery will be used, and what the athletes want to achieve with the imagery. Goals for healing imagery might be to engage in it twice per week to facilitate healing, build confidence, and reduce worry. Goals for soothing imagery might be to do it at the end of each physical therapy session to increase control of pain and ease muscle tension. Goals for performance imagery might involve doing it three times a week, focusing on improving technique and tactics (see Figure 9.2).

Healing

1. _____

2. _____

3. _____

4. _____

5. _____

Soothing

1. _____

2. _____

3. _____

4. _____

5. _____

Performance

1. _____

2. _____

3. _____

4. _____

5. _____

Figure 9.2. Rehabilitation imagery goals. *Note.* From *Psychological Approaches to Sports Injury Rehabilitation* (p. 210) by J. Taylor and S. Taylor, 1997, Austin, TX: PRO-ED. Copyright 1997 by PRO-ED, Inc. Reprinted with permission.

• *Rehabilitation imagery schedule.* After specifying their goals, injured athletes can create a schedule of rehabilitation imagery to achieve those goals. We recommend that they alternate days of healing and performance imagery and include soothing imagery in their physical therapy sessions. Sessions should last about 10 minutes and be done in a quiet place where the athletes can sit or lie in a comfortable position. The sessions should begin with either passive or progressive relaxation to induce a relaxed state that will allow the athletes to be more open to the imagery.

Performance Imagery

Because of its clearly demonstrated benefits, performance imagery is an essential part of the rehabilitation process. Injured athletes should begin their performance imagery program focusing on specific aspects of their sport, such as technique and tactics. Then, as the rehabilitation progresses, they should shift the focus of the imagery to more overall training and competitive performances, culminating with imagery of performances under demanding competitive conditions.

Performance Imagery Ladder

Performance imagery is most effective when it starts at a simple level of performance and evolves through a hierarchy of increasingly more demanding performance situations. The value of this ladder approach lies in enabling injured athletes to incrementally develop their imagery skills and work on their performance goals in progressively more challenging sport scenarios. Injured athletes can begin with the least important and least demanding situation in which they would be performing, for example, a training session, and gradually progress up the ladder to the highest level of performance, for example, an important competition, at the conclusion of their rehabilitation (see Figure 9.3).

Performance Imagery Scenarios

Injured athletes should create specific training and competitive performance scenarios that they can follow in their imagery sessions. These detailed situations should relate to their performance imagery goals, working on, for example, technical, tactical, psychological, or competitive

```
Least Important

1. _____

2. _____

Moderately Important

3. _____

4. _____

Most Important

5. _____
```

Figure 9.3. Performance imagery hierarchy. *Note.* From *Psychological Approaches to Sports Injury Rehabilitation* (p. 214), by J. Taylor and S. Taylor, 1997, Austin, TX: PRO-ED. Copyright 1997 by PRO-ED, Inc. Reprinted with permission.

elements of performance. Injured athletes should use performance-specific imagery. They should clearly identify and generate all relevant aspects of the performance, including setting, participants, level of competition, and weather.

SOCIAL SUPPORT

Athletes often derive part of their motivation to participate in sports from the social aspects of the sport. Athletes gain considerable validation from the friendships they develop and the support they receive while involved in their sport. A particularly difficult aspect of an injury is that they are removed from a significant source of reinforcement, satisfaction, and support.

Social support offers injured athletes a meaningful connection with others that fosters positive emotions, provides encouragement during difficult times, and promotes sharing with others associated with the rehabilitation process, including the sports medicine team, family, friends, coaches, and teammates (Heil, 1993). Social support also ensures that injured athletes have an important means to get necessary information about rehabilitation. It lets them know that they have people to help them to deal with the challenges of rehabilitation.

Social support offers other benefits as well, including improved health, mitigation of stress, increased likelihood of recovery from serious illness or injury (Cohen, 1988; Ganster & Victor, 1988; S. E. Taylor, Falke, Shoptaw, & Lichtman, 1986), greater self-efficacy, and more effective stress management (Sarason, Sarason, & Pierce, 1990). Social support has been inversely related to frequency of injury (Williams & Roepke, 1993) and positively correlated with adherence to rehabilitation (Byerly, Worrell, Gahimer, & Domholdt, 1994; Duda, Smart, & Tappe, 1989). In addition, athletic trainers have indicated that social support is useful for coping with an injury (Wiese et al., 1991) and that they use social support with their patients to facilitate rehabilitation.

Types and Sources of Social Support

Pines, Aronson, and Kafry (1981) suggested that there are two general categories of social support: emotional and technical. Within these two groups, there are six specific types of social support: listening, emotional support, emotional challenge, shared social reality, technical appreciation, and technical challenge. The first four types address the emotional needs of injured athletes and can be given by any individual who is concerned about an injured athlete. The latter two forms of social support involve technical aspects of rehabilitation and the sport in which the injured athlete participates (see Figure 9.4).

The three principal sources of social support for injured athletes are the sports medicine team, teammates, and family and friends (Heil, 1993; see Table 9.2). No one person or group can give all forms of social support to injured athletes. Emotional support can be given by anyone who has a genuine concern for the injured athlete, but family and friends are considered to be the most suitable because of the close ties they have unrelated to the injured athlete's sports participation. Technical support for injured athletes can be credibly given only by individuals who have some expertise in injury rehabilitation and sport, for example, the sports medicine staff, the coaching staff, or teammates (Pines et al., 1981; Rosenfeld, Richman, & Hardy, 1989).

At the start of rehabilitation, injured athletes should be asked whether they feel they are receiving adequate social support, from whom they are receiving it, and how it could be improved. By taking this proactive approach, the rehabilitation team can be sure that social support is facilitating rather than interfering with an athlete's rehabilitation.

Emotional Social Support

Listening—Actively listen without giving advice or making judgments, sharing the joys of success and frustrations of failure.

Example—Listening to doubts and stress expressed by injured athletes about their rehabilitation.

Emotional support—Support an individual during emotionally difficult time without necessarily taking his or her side.

Example—Being present, empathic, and encouraging when injured athletes experience a setback during rehabilitation.

Emotional challenge—Challenge an individual to do his or her best to overcome obstacles and fulfill goals.

Example—Offering motivation and positive challenge to injured athletes faced with obstacles during rehabilitation.

Shared social reality—Others with similar priorities, values, and perspectives who can serve as reality "touchstones," through whom perception of the social context can be verified.

Example—Providing common experiences, emotions, and perspectives on the rehabilitation process.

Technical Social Support

Technical appreciation—Acknowledge when a good piece of work or performance is accomplished.

Example—Reinforcing effort and intensity during a physical therapy session.

Technical challenge—Challenge, stretch, and encourage the athlete to achieve more, to be more creative and excited about his or her work.

Example—Pushing injured athletes to work harder and find new ways to facilitate their rehabilitation.

Figure 9.4. Social support. *Note.* Adapted from "Strategies for Enhancing Social Support Networks in Sport: A Brainstorming Experience," by J. M. Richman, C. J. Hardy, L. B. Rosenfeld, and R. A. E. Callanan, 1989, *Journal of Applied Sport Psychology, 1,* pp. 150–159. Copyright 1989 by the Association for the Advancement of Applied Sport Psychology. Adapted with permission.

Developing a Social Support System

When a rehabilitation social support system is being developed, everyone associated with the injured athlete should be informed about the important role they can play in offering social support. The injured athlete,

TABLE 9.2

Sources of Social Support

Source	Type of Support Provided
Sports Medicine Team	Technical appreciation
	Technical challenge
	Listening
	Emotional support
	Emotional challenge
	Shared social reality (if an athlete has been injured)
Sports Team	Technical appreciation
	Technical challenge
	Shared social reality
Family and Friends	Listening
	Emotional support
	Emotional challenge
	Shared social reality

Note. From *Psychological Approaches to Sports Injury Rehabilitation* (p. 249), by J. Taylor and S. Taylor, 1997, Austin, TX: PRO-ED. Copyright 1997 by PRO-ED, Inc. Reprinted with permission.

however, should take responsibility for actively reaching out to sources of social support. Social support should be a proactive process rather than a reactive one in response to crises (Richman, Hardy, Rosenfeld, & Callahan, 1989).

Rehabilitation Professionals

Rehabilitation professionals have the ability to give injured athletes the greatest variety of social support. Because the rehabilitation team has both long-term and intensive contact with recovering athletes, they can give substantial breadth and depth of support. Moreover, this interaction is very meaningful because it occurs during some of the most difficult times that injured athletes experience, namely, during the pain and stress of physical therapy. The rehabilitation professional is perhaps the only individual in the injured athlete's world who can share the difficult experience and offer both emotional and technical social support. We believe that rehabilitation professionals are natural intuitive psychologists. In

TABLE 9.3

Tips To Enhance Listening Skills

1. Maintain eye contact.
2. Have open body language.
3. Nod head and gesture to show attention.
4. Listen to words and nonverbal message (e.g., emotions, tone of voice, body language).
5. Ask clarifying questions.
6. Allow patient to speak first and to finish.
7. Restate message in your own words.
8. See patient's point of view.
9. Respond to patient's specific concerns.

Note. From "Strategies for Enhancing Social Support Networks in Sport: A Brainstorming Experience," by J. M. Richman, C. J. Hardy, L. B. Rosenfeld, and R. A. E. Callanan, 1989, *Journal of Applied Sport Psychology, 1,* pp. 150–159. Copyright 1989 by the Association for the Advancement of Applied Sports Psychology. Adapted with permission.

other words, their effectiveness comes from both their technical expertise and their ability to respond to the psychological, emotional, and social support needs of the injured athletes with whom they work.

The basis of effective social support is listening (Pines et al., 1981), and rehabilitation professionals appreciate this tool. Athletic trainers believe that listening is an important skill they should learn (Larson et al., 1996; Wiese et al., 1991). Being a good listener allows rehabilitation professionals to obtain useful information about patients that they can use to enhance their rehabilitation while at the same time offering them social support in the form of attentiveness, responsiveness, and caring (Weiss & Troxel, 1986). Table 9.3 offers tips for improving listening skills.

Significant Others

The emotional complications of an injury arise from the physical burden of rehabilitation, the loss of an enjoyable and rewarding activity, and the removal of social support provided through the injured athlete's sports participation. Because the majority of emotional social support comes from significant others such as family and friends (Richman et al., 1989), they should be at the forefront of efforts to create a social support system for the injured athlete. Of the six types of emotional support, family and friends are best able to provide listening and emotional support to injured athletes.

Injured athletes can identify parents, siblings, spouses, and friends who can give them the support they need. These significant others can then be told about the positive impact they can have, the kinds of social support they can provide, and how they can best give this support. The foundation of emotional social support is a positive orientation toward rehabilitation (Fisher, Mullins, & Frye, 1993). Family and friends can build confidence and sustain a positive attitude during difficult periods of rehabilitation when recovering athletes may express doubts about their recovery. This support can bolster commitment to rehabilitation when motivation flags under the tedium and pain of physical therapy and keep recovering athletes focused on progress toward their goal when they have setbacks.

It is not uncommon for significant others to be heavily invested in the sports participation of an injured athlete. This involvement, and the loss due to the injury, can produce feelings of frustration, anger, and sadness in them. If the investment is great and these emotions are strong, they may be communicated to the injured athlete, causing the athlete to not only have to deal with his or her own emotions but also to feel the added responsibility of causing hurt in others close to them. In this case, the family member or friend becomes a burden and a liability instead of a support to help the athlete get through rehabilitation.

Team Rehab

Organizing injured athletes into rehab groups is an effective means of creating social support, teamwork, and a sense of common purpose. For example, the athletic trainer in one junior sports program started Team Rehab, in which team members created a special T-shirt and worked as a group in rehabilitation. Throughout the course of rehabilitation, the group of injured athletes worked together, supported one another, and motivated and pushed one another to recovery. Team Rehab gave them a sense of shared responsibility and commitment to one another and countered the loneliness and separation caused by being away from their sport, thus inspiring them to keep working hard in the face of pain, boredom, and other rehabilitation obstacles (B. Knowles, personal communication, May 2, 1996). Team Rehab provided listening, emotional support, emotional challenge, and shared social reality.

Rehabilitation Support Groups

Rehabilitation support groups give injured athletes a more structured and purposeful setting in which to meet their social support needs (Wiese

& Weiss, 1987). Support groups made up of injured athletes at different stages of recovery provide opportunities for them to both give and receive many types of social support. These groups offer emotional support in terms of perspective on the recovery process and better understanding of the course of rehabilitation from injured athletes who are further along in their healing. Support groups allow injured athletes to express doubts and fears about their injury, to learn that what they are feeling is normal and expected, and to learn from other injured athletes effective ways to cope with the demands of rehabilitation (Granito, Hogan, & Varnum, 1995). Suggestions for establishing a rehabilitation support group include the following (Granito et al., 1995):

- Enlist the support of the sports medicine team.

- Incorporate it into the traditional rehabilitation program.

- Introduce athletes to the support group early in rehabilitation.

- Educate injured athletes about its value.

- Have a member, a sport psychologist, and a rehabilitation professional act as cofacilitators.

- Schedule meetings once a week for a specified time period.

- Provide both support and educational components.

- Choose a weekly topic.

Rehabilitation support groups also give injured athletes technical support in the form of practical information related to progress, pain, setbacks, and logistical functioning that can facilitate their recovery. The psychological benefits from support groups include greater confidence and motivation, reduced worry and stress, and more positive attitude and emotions. Rehabilitation support groups are extremely valuable because they consistently offer all six types of social support—and from individuals with whom injured athletes strongly identify.

Continued Sport Involvement

When athletes are injured, there is usually a practical but unintentional withdrawal from their sport and a loss of contact with their coaches, teammates, and other athletes. Injured athletes, because they are no longer able to fully participate in their sport and must devote their energy to rehabilitation, simply do not have the time to spend on the sport. Teammates and other athlete friends must still devote their time to their sport and often are not able to spend time with an injured athlete. Many athletes also have a superstition that injuries are "contagious" and, as a result, avoid the injured athlete. Coaches also lose touch with injured athletes, because their main focus is on healthy athletes and they simply do not have the time for injured athletes who are not their immediate responsibility. Also, coaches do not generally provide emotional support to their athletes and may not feel that they can offer technical support, so they may not see a role for themselves in supporting injured athletes (Rosenfeld et al., 1989).

Many professionals in the field advocate continued involvement of injured athletes in their sport (e.g., Heil, 1993; Rotella & Heyman, 1993; Williams & Roepke, 1993). The most often used rehabilitation strategy by athletic trainers is to keep athletes involved in their sport (Larson et al., 1996). Injured athletes can continue much of their physical, technical, and tactical training within the limitations of their injury. This sport-specific training can be done in conjunction with the regular training of other athletes. The injured athlete benefits from this participation by receiving support and encouragement from healthy athletes, who in turn may be inspired by the efforts of the injured athlete.

Injured athletes can also stay active in their sport by assuming different responsibilities within the sport. They can help organize various aspects of training and competition, for example, announcing drills, charting competition statistics, and evaluating tactics. This involvement provides them with needed social support, makes them feel like valued and contributing participants, and helps them become more rounded athletes by increasing their understanding of all aspects of their sport.

An essential element of this involvement is the support injured athletes receive from their coaches. The impact that coaches have on injured athletes is greatly underestimated (Rosenfeld et al., 1989). This support is important because injured athletes are more emotionally vulnerable, uncertain of their future ability to perform, and doubtful of their value as athletes. The essential aspect of support from coaches is that it makes athletes feel that they are still valued as athletes and people. In fact, athletic trainers believe coach support of injured athletes is a critical contributor to rehabilitation (Wiese et al., 1991). Discussions with coaches about the role they play with injured athletes is a proactive means of bolstering this valuable support. Encouraging opportunities for regular contact between injured athletes and their coaches can be a worthwhile contribution to the recovery of injured athletes.

REMARKABLE RECOVERY

A compelling aspect of injury rehabilitation is what Heil (1993) termed *remarkable recovery*, which he described as one that is "notable for speediness, for triumph over physical odds, or for movement to a higher level following injury" (p. 148). The timeliness and effectiveness of recovery from an injury depend on a number of physical aspects of the injury, including severity, preinjury physical fitness, individual healing ability, and effectiveness of the rehabilitation program. In addition, Heil suggested that psychological factors can also contribute to the speed and quality of recovery.

Steadman (1982, 1993) found that some injured athletes approach their injury as a learning experience that can help rather than impede their athletic development. He has further stated that some athletes are especially resourceful in their rehabilitation and find new ways to help them deal with their injuries and facilitate recovery, attributing much of their success—as has Heil (1993)—to psychological factors such as goal setting, social support, and overcoming fear of reinjury.

In an attempt to identify some of the psychological contributors to remarkable recovery, Ievleva and Orlick (1991) found that 19% of a sample of seriously injured athletes fit the criteria for "exceptional recovery" (p. 31). They reported that injured athletes who had unusually fast recoveries used positive self-talk, goal setting, and healing imagery significantly more than athletes who had slow or average recoveries. There was also some evidence to suggest that athletes who recovered more quickly were more optimistic, had a more positive attitude, and experienced less stress than those who recovered more slowly. Additionally, athletes who had remarkable recoveries had greater personal control and responsibility for their injury and used more psychological strategies to bolster their recoveries. The exceptional healers were also less fearful of reinjury, and when they did feel some fear, they actively took steps to allay their concerns. Finally, athletes who recovered more quickly indicated that the injury and rehabilitation were valuable learning experiences that enhanced their enjoyment and performance when they returned to their sport (Ievleva & Orlick, 1991). The value of these psychological contributors to remarkable recovery is that they are within the control of all injured athletes and can be used to rehabilitate an injury.

SECTION IV

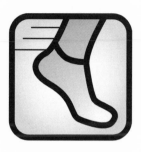

Return
to Sport

CHAPTER 10

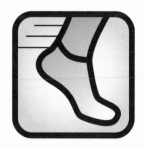

Postrehabilitation Recovery

The end of the structured physical therapy program signals a significant point of transition for injured athletes. This is the time when all of their efforts in rehabilitation are put to the test. Athletes wait for this moment with a conflicting sense of anticipatory excitement at being able to return to their sport and anxious dread that all of the time and energy they put into rehabilitation will have gone for naught.

The perspective that athletes hold and the experiences that they have in their initial return to sport can have a significant impact on their attitude toward the remainder of the return-to-sport process, which in turn can influence the quality of their return to sport and, ultimately, their success in returning as fully functioning athletes. Because of these ramifications, it is essential that sports medicine professionals educate athletes about relevant aspects of the return-to-sport process. Addressing the following concerns can help to ensure that athletes enjoy a healthy return to sport.

- What do full recovery and return to sport mean, and how will I know when I have gotten there?

- What are the physical, psychological, and athletic stages I will go through during my return to sport?

- What kind of progress should I have in my training to attain my previous level of performance?

- What is the likelihood of reinjury, and how can I prevent it?

The answers to these questions are important because, at this point in the recovery process, athletes may be overzealous in their pursuit of a full return to sport. This fervent determination, however well-intentioned, can often lead to a slowed rather than an accelerated return to sport or, at worst, reinjury or injury of a related area. So, a realistic understanding of the return-to-sport process will help athletes recognize the importance of a slow, progressive reentry to sports participation.

WHEN TO RETURN TO SPORT

Return to sport is further complicated by athletes' lack of understanding of what is involved in this process and what is required of them to achieve a full recovery. Despite its importance, this stage of the recovery process is probably the least well defined, and it is often filled with guidelines and ambiguous rules that are not predicated on research, functional outcomes, or evidence-based practice themes. To complicate matters, many factors are involved in the clinical decision-making process about when a patient is ready to return to sport, including the following:

- Chronicity of injury
- Recurrence of injury
- Fitness level of patient
- Presence of injury in areas related to primary injury
- Postural factors
- Type of sport

Chronic injuries, marked by long duration or frequent recurrence, usually entail slow recovery and return to sport. Returning a patient to snowboarding, for example, after five shoulder dislocations would carry greater risks and clinical concerns than would a one-time dislocation. Research has clearly demonstrated the substantial loss of neurological input from the proprioceptive system of the body following an ankle sprain, anterior cruciate ligament (ACL) injury, or shoulder dislocation (Lephart,

Henry, Riemann, Giannantonio, & Fu, 1998; Smith & Brunolli, 1989). Recurrence of such an injury would leave the athlete more vulnerable to further injury because of lack of sensation caused by the neurological deficit. The number of recurrences of an injury also complicates the return process. The process of returning a patient following a first-time shoulder dislocation or ankle sprain usually involves less training and a speedier return program than returning the same patient after numerous episodes of shoulder dislocation or ankle sprain. The cumulative effects of repeated trauma to an area and the subsequent injury of adjacent tissues make the return process more difficult. For this reason, increased effort is always exerted in rehabilitating an initial injury to prevent the negative and cumulative consequences of recurrence.

The fitness level and presence of other injuries further interfere with the rehabilitation and return-to-sport process. Patients may read how, seemingly miraculously, a high-profile elite athlete recovers from a knee arthroscopy in 3 or 4 weeks, not realizing that, coupled with optimal postoperative rehabilitation, the athlete had outstanding preinjury fitness. The injury to adjacent areas may also slow the return process. Following a rotator cuff repair, an athlete with a history or current episode of lateral epicondylitis (tennis elbow) will be slowed in the return process because of the stresses imparted on the adjoining segments.

Other factors of concern in determining a prudent time for return to sport are postural in origin. Individuals with postural deviations such as scoliosis, leg length discrepancies, or severe pronation must take additional care during the return-to-sport process to minimize the effects of these biomechanical factors.

Finally, the type of sport involved is of substantial importance. Returning to a low-impact or physically predictable sport such as golf is far different from returning to gymnastics or basketball, which have unpredictable features. The highest level of preparation and a more complete return of physical capabilities is essential for high-risk sports.

ASSESSING PHYSICAL READINESS TO RETURN TO SPORT

As athletes near the conclusion of the recovery period, there will be many forces exerted on them to return to sport quickly. Family, friends, coaches, and teammates often want the athlete to begin competing sooner than might be wise. The sports medicine team must provide perspective on the risks of starting back too soon and encourage the athlete to look at the long term. Being resolute in the face of pressure from the athlete and others may ultimately determine the quality of the athlete's recovery and return to sport.

Defining physical readiness to return to sport is a critical precursor to starting the return-to-sport program. Many methods can be used to determine full recovery. Most clinicians and sports specialists recommend as much testing as possible. There are two primary types of clinical testing: subjective and objective. Subjective tests are designed to be completed by the patients and typically involve questions aimed at obtaining their perceived level of function. Examples of these tests are listed in Table 10.1. Research has shown that patients can supply consistent information regarding their status across multiple occasions (Beaton & Richards, 1996). Thus, subjective assessment can be a useful part of the overall evaluation of a patient who is approaching the return-to-sport phase of recovery.

Objective testing is performed in several areas to determine the appropriateness of return to sport. Determination of range of motion of the injured joint or joints is carefully performed with a goniometer, or additional flexibility testing can be done using standardized tests like the sit-and-reach maneuver, which measures lower-back and hamstring flexibility. Typically, range of motion equal to the contralateral or uninjured extremity is striven for. Exceptions to matching range of motion to the opposite side might include injury to the opposite side also or presence of exceptional range of motion on one side from playing a unilateral sport such as tennis or baseball. In most patients, however, achieving at least the range of motion of the uninjured side is an appropriate goal.

A determination of strength must also be made before the patient can return to sport safely. Typical strength comparisons use the opposite side as a baseline and employ either manual muscle-testing techniques or more sophisticated equipment like isokinetic or handheld dynamometers that further objectify strength levels and are capable of reliably testing strength at multiple velocities that more appropriately match the speeds at which the muscles and joints function during activities of daily living or some sports activities. Initiation of return-to-sport programs such as running and throwing are not recommended when deficits in muscular strength are 20% or more (Davies, 1992). Although these isolated types of muscle performance tests cannot simulate all functional demands, they

TABLE 10.1
Assessing Physical Readiness To Return to Sport

Type/Name of Test	Common Examples
Subjective Tests	Lysholm (knee)
	Tegner Activity Scale (knee)
	UCLA Rating Scale (shoulder)
	American Shoulder Elbow
	Surgeons (shoulder/elbow)
	Rowe & Zarins (shoulder)
Objective Tests	
Range of motion	Goniometric measurement
	Flexibility tests (e.g., sit and reach)
Strength	Manual muscle testing (MMT)
	Isokinetic muscle testing
	Handheld dynamometer (HHD)
	Repetition Maximum (RM) testing
	(bench press, leg press, squat)
Function	One-leg hop test
	Vertical jump
	Stork standing balance test
	20-yard dash
	Throwing/serving velocity

provide the clinician with a valid indicator of muscular performance around an injured joint.

Additional types of strength testing involve multijoint and multi-muscle group movement patterns that also assess the stability of the rehabilitated area. These are commonly referred to as closed kinetic chain movement or testing patterns. The closed kinetic chain exercise involves a movement in which the end of the extremity is fixed to an object (Palimitier, An, Scott, & Chao, 1991). Examples of closed kinetic chain exercises or movement patterns include squats, StairMaster, and push-ups. These types of muscle performance tests provide valuable insight into the ability of the limb to function as a unit in conjunction with adjoining segments in a functional movement pattern. The disadvantage of this type of closed-chain test is the ability of the muscles around an injured joint to compensate for the injured area and potentially mask a muscular deficit that would otherwise be identified with the more isolated types of muscle testing just described. Therefore, most clinicians recommend combining isolated (also known as open kinetic chain) muscular testing and multiple-joint (closed kinetic chain) muscular testing to more thoroughly test the extremity to determine its readiness for function.

In addition to the objective tests for range of motion and strength, testing specifically designed to assess the function of the rehabilitated area as a whole is recommended. These are typically called functional tests, for example, the one-leg hop and vertical jump, and have been deemed valid for clinical use (Brownstein & Bronner, 1997). One particularly popular test for lower extremity injuries is the one-leg hop test. This test can be performed in a clinic using a tape measure and piece of tape to delineate starting position. The athlete takes off and lands on the same limb, and one limb is compared to the other. Failure to reach the distance generated on the contralateral side may indicate inability to generate gross lower extremity power, as well as hesitancy about landing and having the eccentric control necessary to absorb the load and land on one leg following the jump. Often, patients will land on both legs to protect the injured extremity from the stress and eccentric overload inherent in landing.

Functional tests for the upper extremity are far more limited, with less consensus regarding which is more reliable. One of the commonly used tests is throwing performance (i.e., both speed and accuracy; Davies, 1992). Typical tests such as the number of push-ups in 1 minute or maximal-effort bench press often are not used, because they can cause abnormally high loading patterns to the shoulder joints, as well as the capsule and rotator cuff tendons.

The integration of all components of the evaluation process—including subjective rating scales; objective clinical tests for range of motion, strength, and stability; and functional testing—allows the clinician to determine the athlete's physical readiness for return to sport. Once the clinician establishes that the athlete has achieved minimum levels of competency in the exam areas, it is essential that the athlete not be merely thrown into the sport. This is where the return-to-sport program is employed.

RETURN-TO-SPORT GUIDELINES

One of the biggest mistakes a clinician can make is to give a rehabilitated athlete guidance and guidelines throughout the entire rehabilitation process and then, upon the athlete's discharge from therapy, simply tell the athlete to start playing again. After not performing in their sport for an extended period of rehabilitation, most athletes will likely overdo their initial efforts and exceed their tissue tolerance if strict and concise guidelines are not given.

Warm-Up

Despite the understandable anticipation that an athlete has upon returning to a sport following the hiatus required for injury rehabilitation, a proper warm-up must precede actual performance in the sport. Despite recent evidence that the acute effects of stretching may diminish jump and power performance for a period of up to 20 minutes (Avela, Kyrolainen, & Komi, 1999; Kokkonen, Nelson, & Cornwell, 1998), the potential preventive benefits of warming up make this an important initial stage in all aspects of return-to-sport training. Typically, the warming up consists of a light cardiovascular workout to elevate local tissue temperature and to increase blood flow to the periphery of the limbs (Zachezewski & Reischl, 1986). This warm-up is followed by static stretches with isolated positioning of the muscles' origin and insertion—muscles are moved apart from one another, making the desired muscle stretch—such that controlled and static elongation occurs. Hold times of 15–30 seconds have been reported to produce plastic deformation of the tissue and enhance the flexibility and range of motion of the hamstrings and other muscles (Zachezewski & Reischl, 1986).

In return-to-sport training, passive and active warm-up are recommended. Lower body warm-up typically consists of application of external heat packs if needed, followed by a period of submaximal intensity exercise on a cycle ergometer or treadmill. Upper body warm-up usually consists of an external heat pack if needed, followed by 5–8 minutes on an upper body ergometer. Static stretching of the upper and lower body is used in the warm-up to optimize muscle length and ensure readiness for functional performance.

Aftercare

Equally important as the pretraining warm-up is the aftercare or cooling down following return-to-sport training. In the earlier stages of return to sport, when a physical therapist or athletic trainer is supervising the program, the remainder of a rehabilitation program is typically completed on the same day as the return-to-sport training. Following the sport training, rehabilitation exercises geared at restoring optimal muscle balance, fatigue resistance, joint range of motion, and proprioception are valuable. This allows the athlete to continue developing the injured area during the return-to-sport process.

In the later stages of return to sport, athletes typically perform these continuing maintenance exercises independently of the rehabilitation professional. Strict instructions regarding the amount, intensity, and duration of the maintenance exercises must be shared with the athlete, as well as posttraining stretching and icing. Using ice to create vasoconstriction in the affected area is widely accepted in clinical medicine and sports medicine arenas (Harrelson, Weber, & Leaver-Dunn, 1998). The length of time that ice should be used following a return-to-sport training session has not been formally studied. Current recommendations are typically for application of ice after postworkout stretching for approximately 15 to 20 minutes.

Following an organized and consistent program of aftercare will ensure that off-site continued maintenance efforts mirror the rehabilitation program designed in the clinical setting and is thought to minimize the risk or reinjury and facilitate the return to sport.

Alternate-Day Training Schedule

Athletes who are returning to sport should set up an alternate-day training schedule designed to allow the musculature and static restraint mechanisms surrounding the injured area to recover before resuming sport training. Additionally, the day off following training allows the athletes and the clinician to determine the tolerance of the body to the previous day's level of training intensity. Close monitoring of all subjective symptoms and objective indications is an important part of determining when the next phase of intensity should be initiated.

STAGES OF RETURN TO SPORT

As athletes make the passage from injured athletes to healthy and fully functioning athletes, they will advance through five stages of return to sport: (a) initial return, (b) recovery confirmation, (c) return of physical and technical abilities, (d) high-intensity training, and (e) return to competition. How well athletes progress through the five stages depends on the severity of the injury, the length and effectiveness of the rehabilitation, their postrehabilitation level of physical conditioning, and how much psychological rehabilitation they engaged in. Understanding the five-stage process will make athletes' return to sport seem more achievable and increase their familiarity with and control over what they need to do to ensure a successful conclusion.

The five-stage process relies on the well-known concept of periodization, which is a conditioning program in which systematic alterations are made to the frequency, duration, and intensity of exercise to optimize performance and prevent injury, burnout, or staleness. The periodized model has been studied extensively and its value confirmed in a variety of athletic settings (Fleck & Kraemer, 1986; Roetert & Ellenbecker, 1998). The typical return-to-sport training program following an injury is similar to the periodized training model that has been used to condition athletes for many years.

Initial Return

This initial stage of return to sport is particularly challenging for rehabilitated athletes because it provides the first clear evidence of the success of their rehabilitation. Initial return is essentially an ongoing test of the healed area aimed at reestablishing basic trust, specifically in the rehabilitated area and more generally in the body as a whole. The outcome of this stage will set the overall tone for the remainder of the return-to-sport process. A successful initial return will provide a tremendous sense of relief, build confidence, increase motivation, and create an overall positive atmosphere for the rest of the return to sport. Conversely, difficulties or complications that occur during initial return will negatively affect athletes psychologically and emotionally and create an atmosphere of uncertainty and fear.

As athletes enter the initial return stage of return to sport, they can create unrealistic expectations about how quickly and easily they will make the transition from injured athlete to healthy athlete. We have found that athletes often anticipate that the healed area will be pain-free and they will be able to perform well using it immediately. These expectations can lead to disappointment when they have pain and swelling and their performance is difficult and uncomfortable. These unexpected experiences may produce doubts about the effectiveness of the rehabilitation and raise concerns about the potential success of their return to sport.

The best way to deal with this scenario is to prevent it from occurring by educating athletes about what to expect during their initial return to sport. This approach will ensure that any experiences they have, whether positive or negative, will be viewed as a normal part of return to sport and will facilitate rather than interfere with their progress through return to sport.

A final concern in initial return is the pace at which athletes progress through this stage. In the excitement of having concluded rehabilitation and begun sport training again, athletes can become overzealous and push themselves harder and faster than is safe and prudent. These initially excessive demands can result in reinjury or compensatory injuries that delay rather than accelerate an athlete's return to sport.

To keep athletes' enthusiasm from interfering with good judgment, there should be a clearly defined return-to-sport program, devised in collaboration with the athlete and coaches, that intelligently allows athletes to return to sport as fast as is feasible. The rehabilitation professional should regularly emphasize to athletes that their program was designed especially for them to return to sport in the fastest and safest way possible and that deviation from the plan will put them at risk of slowing their return to sport, as well as sustaining reinjury or new injury. A telling example of this overzealousness is wide receiver Jerry Rice, who returned from a serious knee injury too quickly and, in his first game back, incurred a compensatory injury that kept him out of football even longer (Weiner, 1998).

The emphasis in the initial return phase is to ready the athlete for more intense training. The resistive exercise programming during this phase is one of low resistance with high repetition. This approach is used to promote local muscular endurance and improve blood flow to the injured area (Fleck & Kraemer, 1986). If initial resistance levels are too high, injury may occur and pain levels escalate. Therefore, the high volume and low intensity of training is imperative in this early phase of rehabilitation.

In addition to the resistive exercise used during the initial return phase, emphasis is placed on aerobic and general wellness conditioning. This is an important part of the rehabilitation process when working with an injured athlete. For example, an upper or lower extremity injury can interrupt normal conditioning efforts. With a supervised program from the clinician, aerobic exercise (e.g., on a cycle, in a pool, or using an upper body ergometer) can almost always be included in the early phase of rehabilitation with tremendous physical and psychological benefits to the patient.

Recovery Confirmation

Recovery confirmation occurs at the conclusion of initial return. The purpose of this stage to is clearly confirm to athletes that their injury is fully healed and they are prepared to meet the demands of being a fully functioning athlete. This stage is critical because how successfully they progress through initial return will dictate their attitude about their ability to complete the remainder of their return to sport. If athletes receive confirmation of their recovery, the most significant reaction is one of relief that all of their efforts have paid off and that they are on their way to truly successful recovery and return to sport. This realization bolsters confidence and motivation, relieves stress, and alleviates any other concerns about whether they will recover fully. They are now physically and psychologically prepared for the final, more demanding stages of return to sport.

In contrast, an initial return that involves complications and difficulties can have a dramatically negative effect on the course of return to sport. Athletes have invested considerable time, energy, and pain in their rehabilitation efforts. To have come so far and be forced to admit that their efforts have been for naught can be a traumatic realization. Athletes will question the effectiveness of their rehabilitation and doubt whether they can recover fully. These perceptions will hurt confidence and motivation and, if the problems in initial return were significant enough, may lead to depression or anxiety.

Return of Physical and Technical Abilities

The third stage of return to sport is aimed at athletes' regaining their physical conditioning and technical proficiency. This stage signifies the absolute end of the rehabilitation process and athletes' identification as being injured. From this point forward, they should consider themselves to be healthy athletes in training for their return to high-level performance and competition. Passage through this stage can be facilitated by following many of the recommendations offered throughout this book. These prescriptions include a rigorous physical training program within the constraints of the injury, continued skill development around the injured area, ongoing involvement in the sport, and adherence to a program of psychological rehabilitation. These efforts will reduce "atrophy" of important physical and psychological contributors to return to sport.

In this stage, athletes are ready to apply themselves to a physical and technical training regimen that will prepare them to successfully enter the final two stages of return to sport. Once again, patience should be stressed to the athletes—the return of physical conditioning and technical skills cannot be rushed. Attempts to speed up this process can result in fatigue, illness, or injuries because the body is not yet ready for the demands placed on it. Collaboration with a physical trainer and technical coach in developing an effective training program can ensure athletes' readiness to move to the next stage.

Physical Conditioning

This is one of the most difficult aspects of returning a rehabilitated athlete to sport. The importance of continuing with strength and range-of-motion exercises during the early stages of the return-to-sport process is widely recognized. Restoration of final muscular balance and obtaining the last few degrees of flexibility and motion around a formally restricted joint are all aspects that require continued rehabilitative exercise and conditioning during this phase.

Sport specificity is increased during this phase, in which the rehabilitating athlete performs specific exercises geared at initiating muscular strength, endurance, balance, flexibility, and aerobic conditioning. These important elements prepare the individual for the next phase of the return-to-sport program, which has more specific indications for the athlete's return to sport.

The resistive exercises used during this phase begin to take on more intensity and less volume as athletes are able to build on strength garnered in the initial return phase. Interval training with more intense levels of exertion performed in the subpainful spectrum further challenge the athlete physiologically during this phase. Choosing specific rehabilitation exercises that have more specific or immediate carryover to the athlete's sport is emphasized.

For example, exercises in the initial return phase for an athlete with a rotator cuff injury would be performed with the shoulder in a more neutral (arm near the body) position to minimize the risk or deleterious effects of more overhead positions. In this phase, a more functional position using 90° of elevation in the scapular plane (position used in serving and throwing) would be chosen for an athlete who plays sports that involve overhead motion (e.g., baseball, tennis, basketball). Beginning training with this latter position would likely lead to a violation of tissue tolerance and create injury or irritation in the rotator cuff tendon.

With the foundation of conditioning from the initial return phase, athletes are able to use more aggressive forms of training in the later stages of return to sport. Exercises such as plyometrics, isolated or emphasized eccentrics, and closed-chain functional movement patterns can be safely integrated during this phase. In this stage, the return-to-sport program is coupled with continued maintenance of muscular balance, aerobic conditioning, and muscle power. Sport training and competitive preparation take priority over the ongoing rehabilitation maintenance program. Particular emphasis is placed on finding a balance between maintaining important rehabilitation exercises and not overburdening the athlete with a rehabilitation program that interferes with either return-to-sport training or competitive performance.

The return of full physical conditioning is a progressive process that allows athletes to responsibly increase the demands placed on the rehabilitated area. An example of a progressive conditioning program can be found in the return-to-sport baseball throwing program outlined in Appendix A, which is based on a program developed by Wilk and Andrews (1997). This program involves progressively increasing the volume and distance of throwing based on the position that the athlete plays. This allows for players to continually build strength, flexibility, and stamina in the rehabilitated shoulder.

The return-to-sport tennis program described in Appendix B illustrates how intensity and repetition are progressively increased to develop tolerance to the physical demands of tennis. For example, the rehabilitated player is initially prompted to hit only ground strokes while being fed balls from the net, which produces lower levels of stress to the shoulder and elbow joints, before moving to the more demanding service and overhead motions in later stages of the program. Sequential increases in the intensity of the strokes (e.g., forehands and backhands, then volleys, and finally serves and overheads) allow for a controlled and graduated return to tennis.

Although it is beyond the scope of this chapter to cover every type of return-to-sport program, the foregoing examples show how progressive increases in activity are used to incrementally challenge the healed athlete upon return to sport. The nature of the sport and the particular capabilities of the individual athlete dictate the type of return-to-sport program that is employed. Typically, return-to-sport programs are customized to meet the individual needs of athletes based on previous levels of physical conditioning, severity of the injury, and tissue tolerance. For example, following a shoulder arthroscopy, an athlete would progress faster through a return-to-sport throwing program than would an athlete who had an open surgical repair of a completely torn rotator cuff tendon.

Although there is limited work published in this area, several clinical guidelines are typically followed. Performance of sport-specific activity is recommended prior to any strength training. This is to ensure that the body's musculature, which provides the dynamic stability for the joints, is properly functioning and not fatigued during the functional performance. Additionally, exercises to segments even far away from the injured segment may complicate functional performance. For example, strength training for the trunk or legs is not recommended prior to throwing owing to the important contribution of those segments to power generation during the throwing mechanism (Fleisig, Andrews, Dillman, & Escamilla, 1995). Therefore, return-to-sport training should be performed prior to strength training and other demanding workouts or before the remainder of the rehabilitation exercise program takes place.

Technical Training

Another critical part of the return-to-sport process is the emphasis on proper technique and biomechanics. Returning from an injury can leave athletes with deficits in muscle balance, range of motion, and proprioception in the injured area, which may set the athlete up for compensatory movement patterns. Often these movement patterns can lead to injury in the area being rehabilitated or in adjoining areas. For example, a tennis player returns to play after a knee arthroscopy and develops tennis elbow because of problems with lower body movement and an increase in the contribution and loading on the arm. Another example would be a quarterback returning to throwing after a shoulder injury and, because of a loss in external rotation range of motion, "short-arms" the ball, resulting in greater loading on the inside (medial aspect) of the elbow joint (Marshall, Noffal, & Legnanni, 1993).

Careful monitoring of athletes' mechanics by a coach, a sport biomechanist, or a trained clinician is indicated during return to sport. In most cases, filming the athlete from all sides using a standard video camera and watching the tape with the athlete to allow feedback regarding arm positions, sequential, segmental rotations, and whole-body contributions to force generation can prove invaluable. In some cases, more sophisticated feedback methods can be employed using force platforms, electromyography, and three-dimensional video analysis to monitor force placements, muscle activity patterns, and body segment motions.

It is imperative that the return-to-sport program be discontinued in the presence of compensatory movement activity and potentially harmful sport mechanics. It is better to slow or temporarily halt the return-to-sport process until the athlete has better range of motion, improved strength and endurance, and more normal balance and proprioception than to continue performing the sport and risk further injury.

High-Intensity Training

As athletes enter the high-intensity training stage of return to sport, they should be at or above their preinjury level of conditioning. They should now be fully prepared physically and psychologically to resume their development as athletes. Having established a solid foundation of physical conditioning and technical skills during rehabilitation and in the earlier stages of return to sport, they will now take the final step toward preparing themselves for their return to competition.

The goal of high-intensity training is to expose an athlete's body and mind to the level of demand found in competition. For example, a football running back practices and scrimmages with full contact. In this stage, athletes become reaccustomed to the stresses that they will be required to bear in competition.

At this point in the return-to-sport process, the preinjury capacity of every physical dimension, including strength, stamina, agility, and speed, should be fully regained or surpassed. There should be few indications of the injury other than perhaps a scar, a brace, or some vague sense of the rehabilitated area. Athletes should be psychologically prepared for competition—they should have confidence in their ability to compete again, feel positive and relaxed about competing again, and be totally focused on the final preparations for competition. If athletes had a successful rehabilitation and progressed steadily through the return-to-sport process, they should be physically and psychologically prepared to once again compete at their highest level of performance.

Return to Competition

In their return to competition, athletes experience both excitement at the opportunity to compete again and some concern because it will be the final and most important test of the effectiveness of their rehabilitation. They have many, often conflicting, thoughts and feel a range of positive and negative emotions. These thoughts and feelings may create uncertainty and apprehension.

Therefore, talking to the athletes about their thoughts and emotions, their expectations, and their concerns as their first competition approaches is valuable. It should be emphasized that what they are thinking and feeling is normal and expected. Athletes may place too much significance on the event and become too focused on their success or failure. This attitude can cause stress and distraction, creating discomfort as the date of competition nears and perhaps acting as a self-fulfilling prophecy of poor performance.

Perhaps most important, as athletes prepare for their return to competition, they need to keep the competition in perspective. They should not expect to perform at an outstanding level in their first competitions back from injury. In fact, athletes should have few, if any, outcome expectations. Their primary goal should be to perform comfortably and confidently and to perceive the performance positively in a way that will encourage them to look forward to the next competition. The competition should not be viewed as an all-important event, but rather one small step forward in achieving their athletic goals.

REINJURY

Despite completing all of the stages of a supervised rehabilitation and return-to-sport program, athletes can reinjure themselves, and great care must be taken in dealing with those who do. A thorough physical reevaluation by the physician, physical therapist, and athletic trainer is necessary. Determination of the cause and the extent of the reinjury is of utmost importance. A review of the athlete's supervised and unsupervised rehabilitation and sport training activities will often reveal a violation of the prescribed return-to-sport program in which the athlete was doing too much.

In many cases, minor reaggravation of the supporting structures around an injured joint occurs secondary to overload induced during return-to-sport training. Additionally, failure by the athlete to maintain postrehabilitation levels of muscular strength, balance, endurance, or range of motion is often implicated. Increases in functional sport activity often overshadow the important rehabilitation maintenance program needed to allow the injured area to function at its preinjury level. The lure of increased sport training and reduced rehabilitation and conditioning are often found to be responsible for reinjury.

Members of the sports medicine team play a critical role during this period. The physical therapist or athletic trainer can evaluate and modify the athlete's rehabilitation and conditioning program to heal the reinjury and reduce the likelihood of another reaggravation of the injury. The coach can assess and alter the sport training program to serve the same purpose. The sport psychologist can provide the necessary intervention strategies to allow the athlete to cope with the reinjury or aggravation of the injured area. The sports biomechanist can be consulted to provide more detailed analysis of the athlete's sport activities to prevent further injury and aid in the restorative processes that will be implemented by the rehabilitation team.

Pain and Swelling

Consider an athlete who has just returned to competition. It is about three quarters of the way through a competition, and the athlete is beginning to feel tightness. The area around the injury is starting to get sore. No pain, just tightness and a little swelling. It feels great to be back to full participation for the first time in a long time, but the athlete knows it is not prudent to push it. So the athlete opts out of the remainder of the event and proceeds straight to an ice pack. Does this mean that the athlete is not ready? Did the athlete go back too soon?

The healing process is a complex arrangement of physiological responses that the body must undergo before complete restoration of an injury is achieved. At this later stage in the rehabilitation process, the body is continuing to undergo healing in the form of remodeling and maturation. After the initial stages of inflammation and repair, the remodeling–maturation stage can take as long as a year or more before complete restoration of the injured tissue is obtained. Collagen fibers continue to align themselves in such a way that will ultimately allow for optimal orientation to withstand the forces and increased loads of activity. However, despite adequate healing time, the overall tensile strength of the injured area can be as much as 30% less than that of the original (American Academy of Orthopaedic Surgeons, 1991). This compromised integrity of the damaged tissue contributes to the athlete's low-level symptoms of tightness and residual swelling.

Remodeling Versus Swelling

It is also normal during the remodeling phase for the girth of the injured area to be larger in size—but not due to edema or bleeding. A lot of athletes present with what they perceive as swelling when it is actually a change in the structure of the injured or surgical site. This is why true girth measurements of a joint may not be indicative of underlying pathology. Other factors such as location of perceived swelling, passive and active range of motion, and joint integrity also need to be assessed to ascertain whether there is underlying swelling or inflammation.

Chronic Swelling

For example, an athlete has sustained a moderate sprain of the ankle that has partially torn the anterior talofibular ligament, slightly torn the calcaneofibular ligament, and strained the peroneals and lateral capsule of the ankle. The athlete looks at the ankle, which is moderately swollen, realizes that he or she can limp on it, self-diagnoses it as "tweaked," and decides it should be okay to return to sport within a couple of days. This all-too-common situation is often made worse by a coach or parent with little medical training getting involved and telling the athlete to "tape it up" and keep playing.

What first happens in this situation is that the swelling and edema are never truly brought under control. With the excessive, uncontrolled load to the healing ligaments, a stress response occurs, causing a decrease in the oxygen supply and nutrition to the area. The resultant structural and hormonal changes can cause a cellular response, resulting in chronic inflammation. If care is not taken to reverse these changes, tissue hypoxia and necrosis will occur, making the area more vulnerable to further injury.

Mechanical Dysfunction

Another serious consideration is mechanical dysfunction. Athletes in general move and function in accordance with the demands of the sport and what their body will structurally allow. Put quite simply, structure dictates function. Just as the body's total design often plays a role in deciding which sports and activities athletes might participate in, so too does it have a role in the way the body functions in a sport. Once sports participation is introduced, any subtle mechanical dysfunctions will be significantly exaggerated by increased frequency, intensity, and duration of participation.

Any area of the body that undergoes repetitive stress is vulnerable to subsequent weakening of the affected tissue and potential trauma. There has been a barrage of research on the increased incidence rate of noncontact ACL tears in the female population (Bonci, 1999; Hewett, 1998; Ireland, 1999; Kirkendall & Garrett, 2000; McGee, 1998). Research has also indicated a number of risk factors that may predispose an athlete to this type of injury. Flexibility, posture, hyperlaxity, hormonal effects, notch width, and body position at the time of the injury have all been associated with this increased incidence. One such position, which has been described as the "position of no return" of the knee during movement, is when the pelvis is oriented in an anteriorly tilted position with hip adduction, causing inferior and medial rotation of the femur from proximal to distal end. Subsequent tibial external rotation follows, causing genu valgum, or knock-knee (Ireland, 1999). However, although this was the mechanism of injury, functionally this position is reinforced daily with normal walking and is exaggerated with higher speed, cutting, twisting, and jumping sports (Bonci, 1999; Ireland, 1999; Teitz, Hu, & Arendt, 1997). This can be further complicated if the athlete has an associated navicular drop, severe pronation, or pes planus.

Educating and training athletes during the recovery process about proper joint position—neutral position for all joints—will ultimately decrease the strain on all joints and reduce the risk of reinjury. Research has suggested that controlling the valgus moment at impact when coming down from a jump or when loading the joint excessively, as with cutting and pivoting, can help reduce the number of ACL injuries in women.

Repetitive Stress

One such factor that may affect healing is reducing repetitive low-level stress. For example, an athlete undergoes surgery for chronic shoulder anterior instability. The initial mechanism of injury was a sudden, forceful external rotation of the shoulder joint while the athlete was grasping an opponent's jersey in a basketball game. The athlete had recognized some very low-level symptoms of general soreness after a tough practice or game, but never any real pain or injury. Structurally, the athlete has a very shallow glenoid fossa, stiff and rounded rib cage, and anteriorly oriented scapula, making the inherent function of the ball-and-socket joint less mechanically efficient. The subsequent weakness of the rotator cuff muscles and scapular stabilizers allows for increased joint shear and glide. Postoperatively, the athlete continues to function in the same way as preoperatively. The same stresses from the athlete's general architecture continue to affect the optimal mechanics of the healing shoulder. The anterior aspect of the shoulder gets placed under constant, deleterious stress because of postural considerations.

This is another example of where body awareness and correction of postural and mechanical faults will optimize healing and reduce the risk of reinjury to a healing area. Teaching this basketball player to maintain good, neutral position of all joints as much as possible during the rehabilitation process will not only optimize healing but also reduce the overall pain.

SELF-MAINTENANCE

It is important that athletes recognize the body's limitations and pay heed to them so that nothing is done to exacerbate an injury. Rehabilitation professionals struggle to categorize and develop ways to rule out significant pathology. It is difficult to develop objective measures for pain other than observation. This is the time that athletes need to listen to the warning signs the body may be giving as they are beginning to push the limits. During rehabilitation and return to sport, athletes can learn to distinguish between general awareness of the recovering site, normal soreness at the site, and pain at the site.

There are several useful guidelines for distinguishing significant pathology from expected increased load strain. First, anything that affects athletes' ability to participate in their sport—either psychological or physical—should be considered significant. If athletes recognize it enough that they become preoccupied by it during training and competition, or it is enough to make them change the way they perform (e.g., limping, favoring, compensating), then it should be considered and evaluated. In any case, it would be prudent to wait for those symptoms to subside before full return to sport.

Second, the location of the symptoms should be examined. In surgical cases, for instance, the area that was surgically repaired or stabilized is seldom the cause of any pain or discomfort. It is the area around where the surgery was performed that usually causes the most problems. Being able to differentiate between damage at the repair site, suggesting strain, and damage of surrounding tissue is critical in the decision-making process. Secondary swelling of surrounding bursae or tendons, incision or portal pain, and general capsular or myofascial pain are examples of what could be considered secondary injury symptoms.

A good rule of thumb to follow is the Next Day rule. Any new activity or load should be done by itself and not coupled with other components of the return-to-sport program (e.g., a difficult physical therapy session and practice on the same day). If there is any soreness or swelling at the end of the day, then it should be treated symptomatically with ice and elevation. If the symptoms resolve by the next day, than it most probably was the body adjusting to the increased load. However, if the soreness or swelling continues for a day or two, then it should be assumed that the current physical demands are too great.

BRACING, TAPING, AND SUPPORTIVE DEVICES

In the field of sports rehabilitation, there have been significant advances in the design and function of orthopedic supplies. Although bracing and supportive devices have been used for centuries to treat a host of ailments, it was not until the mid-1900s that they began to play a more prominent role in the rehabilitation process. Taping has become a mainstay in the athletic arena, as have many other types of supportive strapping, bandaging, and bracing devices.

Rehabilitation Braces

Use of braces postoperatively or after significant injury is also a fairly standard practice. The specific diagnosis dictates what amount of support and restriction of movement is indicated, although it is physician preference that determines the model. Again, decisions about what is to be accomplished should play a considerable role in deciding what brand or model to use. Unfortunately, in today's market there are some things that may be out of the physician's control in deciding what brace to use.

Exclusive contracts, financial support for research and programs, and availability are some of the factors that may also dictate which braces are used. Proper application and instruction on using braces are essential for optimizing their value. Also, instructing athletes as to what they are being used for and explaining what particular motions are to be avoided will also improve compliance and efficacy.

Injury Prevention

Prophylactic use of bracing to prevent joint injury—or reinjury—is a practice that can be traced back to Hippocrates. The practice is recorded in the medical literature sporadically over the ensuing centuries. Since the knee derotation brace was first used in football in the 1960s (Cawley, 2000), there has been a significant increase in production of such devices, but with little substantiating evidence of their clinical effectiveness. Although many studies are available on migration, range of motion, neuromuscular changes, and perceived comfort or exertion with prophylactic braces, little is available to determine their true efficacy in preventing deleterious forces on the joint. Most studies aimed at determining true joint stability cannot account for forces exerted during active sports participation.

There are arguments for and against the use of taping or bracing for preventive means in sports. Review of the literature regarding their efficacy or impact on motor control reveals significant inconsistencies. What this research does not account for is the placebo effect and the role it plays in the athlete's *perceived* sense of protective value. Although this psychological benefit may seem to be an invalid reason to use preventive taping, if the athlete is able to perform at an improved level with less apprehension and compensation, then there is value to its use. If a soccer player has a history of minor ankle injuries and is apprehensive about planting and pivoting on that leg, then tape or a supportive brace may make the athlete *feel* more stable and thus less likely to sustain injury. However, prophylactic use of taping or bracing needs to specifically address underlying biomechanical or structural concerns as well. That same soccer player needs to be taped in such a way that the ankle is able to function as normally as possible, while rendering some degree of support. Proper application should account for what and where the anatomical or perceived instability is coming from. Loosely applying tape or a brace, using too many layers of tape, or simply strapping the ankle to restrict normal range of motion is ineffective and may actually predispose the athlete to injury.

If tape or a brace is used, it should be on condition that a specific strengthening and reconditioning program be instituted to address the deficits—whether real or imagined—that the brace is being used to rectify. If an athlete is routinely taped for "weak ankles," the athlete needs a strengthening program for the peroneals, posterior tibialis, intrinsics, and stabilizers. Balance and proprioceptive exercises should be performed as well. An athlete who uses a lateral knee support to decrease the possibility of damage from a lateral blow also needs to do quickness and agility drills aimed at avoidance of catastrophic positions of the knee joint. Making sure that athletes take responsibility for their own conditions and take steps to correct them will further reduce the chance for injury.

Pain Reduction and Neuromuscular Control Improvement

Although braces and taping have been used for years to decrease pain and improve neuromuscular control, only recently have they been used as a primary component in therapeutic intervention of orthopedic injuries. There are a host of different taping and bracing options on the market, with some offering better results than others in achieving the primary objective—optimizing motor function by decreasing pain.

Clinically, it is well established that an athlete should not train or rehabilitate if pain or effusion is present, because this inhibits muscle activity (McConnell, 2000). Taping and bracing techniques have been introduced to reduce pain and optimize motor response, including kinesiotaping, McConnell patella taping (for malalignment, fat pad impingement, or iliotibial band [ITB] syndrome), shoulder taping (for impingement, rotator cuff tendinitis, or bursitis), Mulligan's distal fibula taping (for lateral ankle pain), lateral-medial epicondylitis taping or strapping, and various knee supports. Although there are a number of other products on the market with the same goals, a lot of them have a tendency to negatively affect the mechanics of the joint they are intended to support.

For instance, back supports and braces are often used to decrease back pain and provide support during the injury rehabilitation process. Athletes are usually instructed to use the brace during normal activities of daily living and when performing rehabilitation exercises. What often happens is that athletes become dependent on the brace to hold them in a better posture rather than train their musculature to do the work. Back supports such as these are used to support the back, provide warmth and compression, and remind athletes to maintain correct posture—when they feel the pressure of the brace increase, they should correct their posture. Although sometimes effective at providing pain relief, they often discourage the deep transverse abdominus and multifidi, which are critical for maintaining optimal neutral position, from firing.

There is also a significant debate on whether some of these taping or bracing techniques actually change the mechanics of the area to which they are applied—and even if not, whether they are valid treatment approaches. Several studies, for example, have compared the effects of patella taping and certain patella braces on patella position. Because of the importance of reducing the contact stresses on the patellofemoral joint, and decreasing any incidence of unwanted, increased pressure, other studies have explored whether these techniques actually affect the architecture of the joint. The results have been conflicting as to whether true joint arthrokinematics are altered. The issue for the rehabilitation professional, however, is not whether the tape or brace changes the patellar position, but whether it decreases patients' symptoms by at least 50% so that they can train and compete in a pain-free manner (McConnell, 2000).

Rehabilitation professionals should examine what they are trying to accomplish with the brace and not base their decision on the manufacturer's claims. Using patellofemoral malalignment as an example, for those with true patellofemoral incongruency or a laterally displaced patella—and this should ultimately be determined by Merchant view or skyline X rays—correcting the patella position should be of the utmost concern. Decreasing pain is obviously a goal, but if true arthrokinematics of the joint are left unchanged, then athletes may be putting significant deleterious forces on the knee. With the multitude of braces on the market, all offering different claims as to their effectiveness in correcting patella position, research has shown that only one is truly effective in correcting patella position in the joint during movement (Shellock, Mullin, Stone, & Coleman, 2000).

Stabilization

Using braces and supports designed to provide stability for a joint with increased laxity, or to protect a joint that has previously been injured, is a common practice in sports medicine. The role of braces and supports in providing a mechanical function in the prevention of pathologic motion, their ability to reduce strain to already damaged tissue, and their capacity to augment proprioception and neuromuscular function continue to be defined in the literature. One of the larger impediments in finding conclusive results is lack of sound, long-term outcome data—especially for the knee. There are stabilizing braces for every major joint in the body and, depending on the amount of laxity and the inherent design of the joint (i.e., hinge vs. ball-and-socket), they provide some level of protection in decreasing shear and rotational forces on the joint.

Wojtys, Kothari, and Huston (1996) compared the effects of six different functional knee braces on anterior tibial translation, isokinetic performance, and neuromuscular performance on ACL-deficient knees. For anterior tibial translation, they compared the effects with and without brace use and with and without muscle response, as monitored by electromyogram. Isokinetic performance was measured with and without brace use as well. They found that braces decrease anterior tibial translation between 28% and 39% without the stabilizing contractions of the quadriceps, hamstrings, and gastrocnemius muscles. With the introduction of lower extremity muscle activation, the stabilizing effects of the brace increased to 69%–84%. However, isokinetic testing found that with brace application, most of the braces consistently slowed hamstring muscle reaction times.

The effects of stabilizing braces were also studied by Ashton-Miller, Ottaviani, Hutchinson, and Wojtys (1996). They compared the effects of different ankle braces, taping, and supportive shoes, as well as neuromuscular response, on the ability to stabilize the ankle at the inversion moment. Biomechanical calculations suggested that at 15° of inversion, the ankle evertor muscles isometrically developed a moment six times greater than that obtained by wearing a three-quarter top shoe and up to three times greater than that obtained using tape or a supportive brace. They concluded that the strength and motor response of the ankle evertor muscles were the best protection for a near-maximally inverted ankle at foot-strike.

Both of these studies reach the same conclusion: Braces can be effective in controlling forces on an injured area, but neuromuscular response as indicated by proprioception and muscle firing patterns is superior for the ultimate stability of a joint. Braces can be an effective tool in *helping* provide stability to an area, but specific rehabilitation exercises aimed at improving motor control should be continued as long as the athlete wears a supportive device.

Again, application of the brace is of the utmost importance as well. Common sense dictates that if a brace is properly fitted, then it will have the best effect on stabilizing the area. However, many athletes who wear braces either apply them improperly (i.e., not optimally aligned to the joint), or migration and slippage occur during athletic performance and proper refit is never achieved. Proper instruction on fitting any brace based on manufacturer's guidelines is essential. So, too, is educating the athlete that if the brace moves at all, then it should be completely refitted and not just pulled back up into place.

POSTREHABILITATION PHYSICAL THERAPY

Because of recent changes in the health care system in the United States, athletes rehabilitating from orthopedic injuries frequently have rehabilitation needs that exceed the authorized or available visits for formal physical therapy. These changes have produced a dilemma among athletes, rehabilitation professionals, and physicians. Current practices among American athletes is to utilize rehabilitative care provided by their insurance carrier only, with additional self-payment visits seldom arranged. This trend, coupled with the limited number of visits allowed by insurance carriers for orthopedic injury, surgery, or rehabilitation, has required creative or alternative programming by rehabilitation specialists.

One creative and increasingly popular option is postrehabilitation training programs, which evolved to bridge the gap between formal, supervised physical therapy and independent home- or gym-based exercise programs. Research demonstrates limited compliance by patients with traditional orthopedically based exercise programs. Exercise compliance was found to substantially decrease as the number of exercises increased. This severely limits the ability of rehabilitation professionals in providing a comprehensive home-based rehabilitation program. Postrehabilitation training programs typically involve extended use of the physical therapy location where supervised rehabilitation was taking place.

In many cases, modality care and most aspects of hands-on care are not required at the time of transition of athletes to the postrehabilitation training program. The postrehabilitation training program is offered primarily to allow athletes to use the equipment and familiar exercise procedures that they have become acquainted with during formal rehabilitation. The confidence inherent in continuing a self-directed rehabilitation program in the same setting as formal rehabilitation is one of the benefits of the postrehabilitation training program. Additional benefits are the availability of continued limited supervision and interaction with rehabilitation professionals, as well as an element of accountability that cannot be replicated with a completely home-based rehabilitation program.

Examples of injuries that frequently benefit from this type of postrehabilitation training program are completely torn ACL and rotator cuff and lumbar spine dysfunction. Some of the beneficial elements for ACL reconstruction include progression of closed-chain and functional lower body exercises, isokinetic training, balance and perturbation training, and lower impact cardiovascular training. Rotator cuff repair benefits from exercise equipment that facilitates rotator cuff muscle strength and endurance, such as internal and external rotation machines, cable pulleys with lighter and more graduated weights than those found in most health clubs, as well as upper body ergometers and isokinetic training. Finally, lumbar rehabilitation benefits from the stabilization equipment and cardiovascular machines, which are not often found in traditional health club settings.

The postrehabilitation training program provides athletes and the rehabilitation staff with a continuum of care. It progresses from the initial evaluation with closely monitored and supervised manually based exercise and joint mobilization, to less supervised and more independent training geared at achieving more complete levels of strength, endurance, and flexibility following an injury. Typical application of postrehabilitation training programs follows an alternate-day training schedule. Days of recovery are interspersed between training sessions similarly to most current rehabilitation programs in the outpatient setting. Although not all rehabilitation centers provide this service, many outpatient facilities have adopted the system or a variation thereof. The presence of such a program should be marketed; it clearly identifies rehabilitation facilities that are making an important effort to provide this continuum of care for their patients.

Discharge of the patient from the postrehabilitation program must be accompanied by formal instruction in a continued program that is home or health club based. This final effort by the rehabilitation professional ensures that athletes are guided toward a continued and often lifelong modification of activity, complete with an integrated exercise program that continues to address full functional return of the formerly injured area. The postrehabilitation training program is not meant to replace the home program or compete with the traditional weight room or health club program. Rather, this program can be optimally used as a transition from rehabilitating athlete to fully functioning athlete by allowing for a continuation of appropriately guided rehabilitation care until athletes are cleared to cease supplemental rehabilitation training.

CHAPTER 11

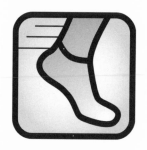

Psychological Concerns of Return to Sport

An emphasis throughout this book has been on the role that psychological issues play in the quality of injury management that athletes experience. This influence is no less important as athletes reach the end of their recovery. It must be appreciated that athletes will be participating in the sport in which they were injured. Moreover, it might have been many months since the injury. Therefore, a variety of psychological and emotional concerns is normal and expected. These concerns are heightened because athletes do not truly know whether their rehabilitation has been successful and the injury is behind them until they are able to perform at or above the preinjury level.

Sports medicine professionals can give athletes the information and psychological tools they need by addressing the following concerns:

- How can I regain confidence in my sport when the last time I performed I got injured?

- What can I do to allay my fear of reinjury?

- How do I make sure my intensity helps rather than hurts me as I return to my sport?

- How do I block out all of those irrelevant distractions and stay focused on performing my best?

- What mental skills can I use to make my return to sport better?

The sports medicine team typically has little contact with the athlete during this final stage of injury management. However, addressing these issues at the end of formal rehabilitation and providing some ongoing follow-up in response to the diverse concerns that often arise can ensure that athletes are prepared for and successfully arrive at the conclusion of the sports injury management process.

IMPORTANCE OF RETURN TO SPORT

As rehabilitated athletes enter the return-to-sport phase of the injury management process, they are faced with myriad thoughts and emotions, ranging from excitement that their injury is behind them to doubts that they will be able to perform at their preinjury level. At this point, rehabilitated athletes are finally going to find out whether all of their efforts will pay off in a full return to sport.

One factor that influences the effectiveness of their return to sport is whether their attitude is one of threat or challenge. A threat response has many negative influences that interfere with return to sport. Most basically, athletes who have a threat response move away from difficult aspects of return to sport to avoid having to face the potential failure. Signs of a threat response include comments about not being ready to return, complaints of instability, unsubstantiated pain, and reduced adherence to their rehabilitation regimen. Particular problem areas that are evident are low confidence, reluctance or resistance to return, stress, and a negative outcome focus.

Athletes who view their return to sport as a challenge present an entirely opposite set of responses, beginning with an attitude in which return to sport is looked forward to and sought after. Indications of a challenge response are a positive attitude, high motivation to return, enthusiasm, and a process focus.

Prevention is the best way to deal with possible threat responses in returning athletes. Using the information and techniques advocated in this book to facilitate injury management can lessen the likelihood that a threat response will occur. However, despite efforts to prevent a return-to-sport threat response, some athletes will have difficulties during the transition from rehabilitation to full sport participation.

Discussion of these issues with athletes as they approach return to sport can allay many of their concerns and provide them with a positive, realistic, and healthy perspective as they enter this crucial final stage of injury management. These conversations can also benefit athletes by showing them that what they are thinking and feeling is a normal and expected part of the return-to-sport process. Athletes can also become so focused on their ambivalent feelings about their return to sport that they forget why they have worked so hard to rehabilitate, the importance of a complete return to health and participation in their sport, and their commitment to renewing and surpassing their previous level of performance.

RETURN-TO-SPORT CONFIDENCE

Confidence is the most significant psychological concern as athletes enter their return to sport. Return-to-sport confidence often determines whether athletes perceive return to sport as a threat or a challenge. It derives from their efforts in their physical and psychological rehabilitation and is influenced by how they progress through the return-to-sport process. Physical and psychological experiences that athletes had during their rehabilitations and that they will have during their return to sport will either foster or inhibit their confidence as they approach the final stages of their return to sport.

The foundation of return-to-sport confidence is the belief that the injured area is now fully rehabilitated and healed and that the athlete is at a high level of physical conditioning and can return to a high level of competitive performance. The basis for this confidence lies in an effective rehabilitation program that maintains and enhances relevant physical areas that influence return to sport. It also depends on developing the important psychological areas that bear on rehabilitation and return to sport (as discussed in Chapters 8 and 9). Active use of these strategies will ensure that the athlete has the return-to-sport confidence to effectively proceed to the end of the injury management process.

Return-to-sport confidence is also affected by how the athlete proceeds through the return-to-sport process. A progression that is consistent and builds on small successes will increase confidence steadily with few declines. A process that is too fast and in which the athlete has regular setbacks will hinder confidence and slow the athlete's return to sport.

FEAR OF REINJURY

It is often thought that the conclusion of rehabilitation is also the end of concerns for psychological distress in athletes. Yet, fear of reinjury can be one of the most significant sources of distress in the return-to-sport process (Heil, 1993). Fear of reinjury comes from the athlete's belief that healing was not complete and that he or she is not prepared to effectively return to sport. Fear of reinjury can negatively affect return to sport psychologically by lowering confidence and causing interfering distractions and physically by producing muscle tension and bracing and hurting coordination.

The prevention and treatment of fear of reinjury is an ongoing and intrinsic part of every rehabilitation program and includes every physical and psychological strategy that is used during rehabilitation. All efforts during rehabilitation are directed toward developing in athletes complete confidence in their ability to return to their sport at or above their previous level of performance, with no doubts, worry, or hesitation caused by concern of reinjury. Table 11.1 provides guidelines for preventing reinjury.

Causes of Fear of Reinjury

The most basic cause of fear of reinjury is an incomplete recovery or the perception that rehabilitation was ineffective. The former problem is exacerbated when there are measurable decrements in physical parameters associated with the injury. In this case, the concern for reinjury is legitimate, and serious consideration should be given to delaying the start of the return-to-sport phase of injury management. The belief that rehabilitation was not effective can be just as debilitating. These doubts can be caused by complications or setbacks that slowed rehabilitation. Because of these problems, athletes may question how well they have healed and how prepared they are to return to sport. This lack of confidence in the injured area affects athletes physically and psychologically, not only causing fear of reinjury but also increasing the chances of reinjury when they return to their sport.

Fear of reinjury can also be caused by overzealousness of athletes to return to sport. In their impatience, they may do too much too soon, placing demands on their body that, because of the long layoff, it was not

TABLE 11.1
Patient Education Guide: Preventing Reinjury

1. Ensure high level of overall physical conditioning before return to sport. Get in shape to play the sport; do not play the sport to get in shape.
2. Follow the interval return-to-sport program closely. Be patient!
3. Continue rehabilitation home exercises after return to sport until cleared by sports medicine professional.
4. Have biomechanics evaluated by a coach or sport biomechanist.
5. Incorporate rest days in return-to-sport training to prevent overtraining.
6. Progressively build confidence and trust by successfully placing increasingly greater demands on the rehabilitated area.
7. Use relaxation exercises if anxiety is present before and during sport training.
8. Focus on sport-relevant cues rather than on the formerly injured area during training.
9. Stretch before and immediately following sport training.
10. Ice injured area after sport training to control inflammation or re-aggravation.
11. Listen to your body. Be responsive to injury-site pain (do not try to work through it).

ready to handle. This eagerness then results in reinjury of the formerly damaged area or compensatory injury of a related area. These physical difficulties negatively affect athletes psychologically as well, hurting confidence, increasing stress, causing distractions, and further reinforcing fear of reinjury. Their impatience can also lead to performance setbacks because they may not be prepared for the demands of competition. This entire scenario slows return to sport rather than achieving the intended desire to speed it up.

Fear of reinjury can also be triggered by the nature of the sport. Sports that have inherent risks, such as soccer, gymnastics, and wrestling, involve athletes' returning to a sport in which they were injured the last time they participated. These concerns are legitimate and must be recognized and responded to.

Prevention of Fear of Reinjury

A significant means of prevention of fear of reinjury is keeping rehabilitating athletes actively involved in their sport. Fear of reinjury can be deepened by the disconnectedness that results while athletes are re-habilitating. The physical and emotional distance that occurs produces a generalized feeling of discomfort and a loss of familiarity with the sport setting when they return. To combat this effect, injured athletes can take on responsibilities in training and competition. They can also work on technique and physical conditioning unrelated to the injured area.

Fear of reinjury can also be prevented by having injured athletes come to see rehabilitation as athletic performance. With this perspective, athletes are able to regularly place the injured area under stress in the form of rehabilitation. It also allows them to practice their psychological, training, and competitive skills in rehabilitation, thereby keeping them honed for their return to sport.

Full participation in their sport is not possible while athletes are rehabilitating an injury, but they can still perform at their highest level using performance imagery. Performance imagery enables athletes to continue to perform in their sport by seeing and feeling themselves in training and competition (see Chapter 9). There is considerable evidence to support the effectiveness of mental imagery in enhancing athletic performance (for a review, see Suinn, 1993; Vealey & Walter, 1993), and it can be a valuable technique for maintaining and develop-ing psychological, technical, and competitive skills while recovering from injury.

Perhaps the most important way to prevent fear of reinjury is a timely, disciplined, and steady return to sport when the sports medicine staff fully clears the athlete to resume sports participation. This progres-sive approach enables athletes to slowly expose the rehabilitated area and the athletes' mind and body in general to incrementally greater demands in training. With successful early experiences in return to sport, athletes can regain trust that they are once again ready for high-level training and competition. This encouragement increases confidence and lessens fear of reinjury.

Treatment of Fear of Reinjury

Although prevention of fear of reinjury will reduce the likelihood of its interfering with return to sport, some athletes will still experience some difficulties. Particularly as athletes regain the role of fully functioning participants in their sport, fear of reinjury may arise and should be dealt with immediately. Athletes should understand that some fear of reinjury is normal and expected. The last time they participated in their sport, their body did not meet the demands placed on it, so a degree of mistrust is natural. This fear usually passes as athletes reacquaint themselves with their sport and they remember what it feels like to perform again.

Some fear of reinjury may simply be a phase that athletes pass through, but it is best to take a proactive approach to ensure that the fear is allayed as soon as possible so that it does not interfere with the return-to-sport process. As a first step, the cause of the fear should be identified. The situation that tends to trigger a strong fear reaction is the first time athletes are put in the situation in which they were injured. Once the cause is specified, athletes can be shown that a similar injury is less likely now for a variety of reasons. For example, new equipment decreases the likelihood of the injury, or the athlete is much stronger than before the injury.

Athletes must also learn through direct experience, progressively performing again in that situation. Athletes should start out performing at 50% intensity and speed and as they become more comfortable steadily increase the intensity and speed to 100%. Each successful experience in this progression reaffirms to athletes that the healed area is once again capable of sustaining itself under the demands of performance.

RETURN-TO-SPORT FOCUS

A significant challenge for rehabilitated athletes when they return to sport is redirecting their focus, which has been preoccupied with the injury, onto cues that will facilitate their return to full functioning and sports participation. For example, in one case a junior tennis player who sustained a third-degree sprain of her right ankle was so focused on her injury when she returned to the court that she could not move well or hit the ball the way she wanted to. Her injury focus was distracting her from paying attention to relevant cues for tennis, it was hurting her confidence because she was playing poorly, and all of these things were putting her under considerable stress. Interfering foci can be physical, technical, social, or psychological, and each can hinder the return-to-sport process.

Physical Distractions

The most salient physical distraction for rehabilitated athletes is a fixation on the formerly injured area. If athletes are preoccupied with the area, they are not focusing on important performance cues. This negative focus not only will hurt performance but also will increase the likelihood of risk of reinjury. It can be useful in establishing effective return-to-sport focus for athletes to identify cues that are interfering and cues that will enhance performance to make them more aware of when they are focusing poorly.

Poor overall physical conditioning can be another physical distraction when athletes enter the return-to-sport phase of injury management. In serious injuries requiring lengthy rehabilitation, athletes most often are not immediately ready for intense training. This perception of poor fitness can result in concern with their lack of readiness to return to sport. When this belief is combined with a preoccupation on the healed area, athletes can be physically and psychologically vulnerable to reinjury or a new injury.

Three steps can be taken to relieve this interfering physical focus. As a means of prevention, athletes should participate in a strenuous general physical conditioning program to minimize decline in conditioning and to maintain confidence in their physical ability. At the conclusion of rehabilitation, time should be allotted for athletes to regain a level of conditioning necessary to handle the stresses of return-to-sport training. Ultimately, the only way to attain a performance-ready level of fitness is by participating in the sport. So an incremental return that will allow athletes to progressively regain the required level of conditioning and enable them to shift their focus away from physical concerns and onto performance is best (Pollard, 1994).

Technical Distractions

A particularly frustrating aspect of return to sport for athletes is the difficulty of regaining their technical skills, especially after a lengthy recovery in a technically demanding sport such as basketball or golf. Skills that were once automatic can, upon return to sport, seem unfamiliar and uncomfortable. Because of this discomfort, athletes can become preoccupied with the minutiae of technique and lose sight of the overall execution of the skills in the process of performance. This absorption in technique can cause other focusing problems. Athletes who are focused on the specifics of technique are not attending to more general performance cues. For example, a soccer player focusing too much on his footwork following a knee injury may not pay enough attention to the action on the field.

This preoccupation with technical details can also interfere physically and psychologically. It can cause muscular bracing and a loss of flow, which leads to frustration from not feeling comfortable and a decline in confidence at not being able to perform well. This cycle can in turn create stress, increase the risk of reinjury, hurt performance, and interrupt the return-to-sport process.

As with many of these issues, prevention can avert most technical distractions before they arise. One problem with an injury is that athletes become removed from their sport and lose touch with many potentially beneficial aspects of their sport, including technical development. Technical skills can be sustained and also improved during recovery from an injury. One way to maintain technical skills is by watching the sport live or on video during rehabilitation. Observing other athletes can help keep the images and feelings of performing fresh and familiar.

Technical skills can also be improved during rehabilitation. Contrary to many injured athletes' perceptions that they will automatically fall behind in their technical development, rehabilitation can be a period in which technique is not only maintained but also honed. For example, a basketball player with a broken dominant right hand was able to improve her dribbling with her left hand while she waited for her injury to heal. When she returned to playing, she was a better overall basketball player because of her injury. Finally, as discussed in Chapter 9, performance imagery that emphasizes technique and execution can also facilitate maintenance and development of technical skills.

Athletes can decide what technical skills they can realistically practice during rehabilitation. They can then use physical practice, observation, and performance imagery throughout their recovery to maintain and further their technical development. Athletes who use this approach should be able to perform technically with comfort and smoothness, focus better on the overall aspects of performance, and progress more easily from rehabilitation to return to sport.

Social Distractions

Social distractions during return to sport are perhaps the most difficult to deal with because they are outside athletes' control. They consist of attention that athletes receive when they return to sport, renewed expectations from others, and pressure to return to competition quickly. Social distractions can come from family, friends, coaches, teammates, and, in the case of high-profile athletes, from media and fans. A survey of collegiate female volleyball players indicated that almost one quarter of them felt pressure to return from their coaches (Gipson et al., 1989).

Because social distractions are not directly controllable, the only way they can be relieved is to remove the source of the distraction. This can be accomplished by identifying the source of the social distraction, communicating with that person or persons about how their behavior is interfering with rather than encouraging an effective return to sport, and hoping they are responsive enough to stop the distraction. This approach will be effective only if the source of social distraction has a genuine and well-intended interest in the returning athlete and wants to do what is best for the athlete.

Unfortunately, many people who become social distractions have an agenda other than the best interest of the athlete. In these cases, the emphasis must be on athletes' learning to distance themselves from the distractions physically or emotionally. The most direct means of dealing with social distractions is to avoid them. If athletes are not around these people, they will have little or no impact on their focus. For example, a high school running back recovering from ACL reconstruction felt pressure from the school's athletic director to play against the school's intrastate rival in a game at the end of the season. This pressure was most often felt when he walked by the athletic director's office on the way to the training room. The player's solution was simple; he took another route to physical therapy.

Psychological Distractions

Psychological distractions can be a significant obstacle to return to sport. It is natural for recovered athletes to question whether they can return to their preinjury level of performance and to feel some anxiety about putting the injured area to the test. An important objective of early return to sport is to allay those doubts and relieve any anxiety they may feel.

It is not unusual, however, for some athletes to become preoccupied with doubts and negative thoughts to the detriment of effective performance. This negative focus keeps them from attending to relevant performance cues and causes hesitancy that hurts performance and increases the risk of reinjury. The likelihood of psychological distractions interfering with return-to-sport performance can be largely averted by using the psychological rehabilitation techniques discussed in Chapter 8. These strategies can be used during rehabilitation and return to sport to increase confidence, reduce stress, direct focus, and facilitate renewed performance.

Achieving Return-to-Sport Focus

Being able to focus properly on performance-relevant cues during return to sport is essential for regaining preinjury form and performance (Pollard, 1994). Achieving and maintaining focus begins with identifying facilitating and interfering cues that athletes will face upon their return to sport. Potential interfering internal cues include preoccupation with the injured area, fixation on technique, and negative thinking. Interfering external cues include concern over who is watching or what others are saying about the athlete. This understanding will enhance athletes' awareness of ineffective focus and their ability to recognize poor focus when it occurs in the early stages of return to sport.

Athletes can then specify technical, tactical, physical, and psychological cues that will help performance. They can choose two or three cues to focus on that are most relevant to what they are doing at their current stage of return to sport. For example, a collegiate softball pitcher recovering from a second-degree shoulder separation might focus on being relaxed and keeping a long and loose pitching motion.

RETURN-TO-SPORT IMAGERY

Return-to-sport imagery is another valuable tool for making the transition to fully functioning athlete. Although healing and soothing imagery are most useful early in the injury management process, performance imagery focused on return to sport is most critical as athletes approach the conclusion of their rehabilitation. The value of return-to-sport imagery is that it enables athletes to practice their reintroduction to sport training and performance before they actually begin the process. This imagined rehearsal generates successful images and feelings that enhance familiarity and comfort, increase motivation to return to sport, bolster confidence, create a constructive focus, and foster positive emotions associated with return to sport. Adding relaxation techniques (described in Chapter 9) before beginning return-to-sport imagery can further facilitate this process by inducing a positive physical state to accompany the positive images, thoughts, and emotions.

APPENDIX A

Return-to-Sport Throwing Program for Baseball Players

The Return-to-Sport Throwing Program (RSTP) was designed to gradually return motion and strength to the throwing arm after injury or surgery by slowly progressing through graduated throwing distances. The RSTP is initiated when the athlete's physician gives clearance for the patient to resume throwing and is performed under the supervision of the rehabilitation team (physician, physical therapist, and athletic trainer). The program is set up to minimize the chance of reinjury and emphasizes prethrowing warm-up and stretching. The following factors are considered most important in developing the interval throwing program:

- The act of throwing the baseball involves the transfer of energy from the feet through the legs, pelvis, trunk, and out the shoulder through the elbow and hand, so any return to throwing after injury must include attention to the entire body.

- The chance for reinjury is lessened by a graduated progression of interval throwing.

- Proper warm-up is essential.

- Most injuries occur as the result of fatigue.

- Proper throwing mechanics lessen the incidence of injury and reinjury.

- Baseline requirements for throwing include pain-free range of motion of all joints involved in throwing, adequate muscle power, and resistance to fatigue.

Because the amount of time it takes for individuals to recover from injury varies, there is no set timetable for completion of the program. Most athletes, by nature, are highly competitive individuals and wish to return to competition as soon as possible. However, proper channeling of the athlete's energies to a rigidly controlled throwing program is essential to lessen the chance of reinjury during the rehabilitative period. Athletes tend to want to increase the intensity of the throwing program. This increases the incidence of reinjury, however, and may greatly retard the rehabilitation process. Following the program rigidly will be the safest route to return to competition.

During the recovery process, the athlete will probably experience soreness and a dull, diffuse aching sensation in the muscles and tendons. If the athlete experiences sharp pain, particularly in the joint, all throwing activity should cease until this pain ceases. If pain continues, the physician, physical therapist, or athletic trainer should be contacted.

WEIGHT TRAINING

The athlete should supplement the RSTP with a high-repetition, low-weight exercise program. Strengthening should address a good balance between anterior and posterior musculature, so that the shoulder will not be predisposed to injury. Special emphasis should be given to posterior rotator cuff musculature for any strengthening program. Weight training will not increase throwing velocity, but it will increase resistance of the arm to fatigue and injury. Weight training should be done the same day as throwing, but it should be after throwing is completed, using the day in between for flexibility exercises and recovery. A weight-training pattern or routine should be stressed at this point as a "maintenance program." This pattern should be maintained by the athlete into and throughout the season as a deterrent to further injury.

INDIVIDUALIZED RSTPs

The RSTP is designed so that each level is achieved without pain or complication, before the next level is started. This sets up a progression in which a goal is reached prior to advancement, instead of advancing according to a specific time frame. Because of this design, the RSTP may be tailored to meet the needs of individuals with different levels of skills and abilities, from those in high school to professional levels. The following are general guidelines for all individuals:

• *Warm-Up.* Jogging increases blood flow to the muscles and joints, thus increasing their flexibility and decreasing the chance of reinjury. Because the amount of warm-up needed varies from person to person, the athlete should jog until developing a light sweat, then progress to the stretching phase.

• *Stretching.* Because throwing involves all of the muscles in the body, all muscle groups should be stretched prior to throwing. This should be done in a systematic fashion, beginning with the legs and including the trunk, back, and arms. It should be followed by capsular stretches for the shoulder, particularly the posterior capsule, and range of motion for the elbow and wrist.

• *Throwing Mechanics.* A critical aspect of the RSTP is maintenance of proper throwing mechanics throughout the advancement. Use of the "crow-hop" method simulates the throwing act, allowing emphasis on proper body mechanics. This throwing method should be adopted from the onset of the RSTP. Throwing flat-footed encourages improper body mechanics, placing increased stress on the throwing arm and, therefore, predisposing the arm to reinjury. The pitching coach and sports biomechanist (if available), with their knowledge of throwing mechanics, can be valuable allies to the rehabilitation team. Additionally, video analysis of throwing mechanics can help ensure proper throwing mechanics and provide valuable feedback to the athlete. Components of the crow-hop method are, first, a hop, then a skip, followed by the throw. The velocity of the throw is determined by the distance, whereas the ball should have only enough momentum to travel each designed distance.

• *Throwing.* Using the crow-hop method, the athlete should begin warm-up throws at a comfortable distance (approximately 30–45 feet) and then progress to the distance indicated for the particular phase the athlete has reached (see Table A.1). The object of each phase is for the athlete to be able to throw the ball without pain the specified number of feet (45, 60, 90, 120, 150, 180) 75 times at each distance. After the athlete can throw 180 feet 50 times without pain, he or she will be ready for throwing off the mound or return to his or her respective

TABLE A.1

Return-to-Sport Throwing Program for Baseball Players

45-Foot Phase

Step 1

1. Warm-up throwing
2. 45 feet (25 throws)
3. Rest 15 minutes
4. Warm-up throwing
5. 45 feet (25 throws)

Step 2

1. Warm-up throwing
2. 45 feet (25 throws)
3. Rest 15 minutes
4. Warm-up throwing
5. 45 feet (25 throws)
6. Rest 10 minutes
7. Warm-up throwing
8. 45 feet (25 throws)

60-Foot Phase

Step 3

1. Warm-up throwing
2. 60 feet (25 throws)
3. Rest 15 minutes
4. Warm-up throwing
5. 60 feet (25 throws)

Step 4

1. Warm-up throwing
2. 60 feet (25 throws)
3. Rest 15 minutes
4. Warm-up throwing
5. 60 feet (25 throws)
6. Rest 10 minutes
7. Warm-up throwing
8. 60 feet (25 throws)

90-Foot Phase

Step 5

1. Warm-up throwing
2. 90 feet (25 throws)
3. Rest 15 minutes
4. Warm-up throwing
5. 90 feet (25 throws)

Step 6

1. Warm-up throwing
2. 90 feet (25 throws)
3. Rest 15 minutes
4. Warm-up throwing
5. 90 feet (25 throws)
6. Rest 10 minutes
7. Warm-up throwing
8. 90 feet (25 throws)

(continues)

TABLE A.1. *Continued.*

120-Foot Phase

Step 7	Step 8
1. Warm-up throwing	1. Warm-up throwing
2. 120 feet (25 throws)	2. 120 feet (25 throws)
3. Rest 15 minutes	3. Rest 10 minutes
4. Warm-up throwing	4. Warm-up throwing
5. 120 feet (25 throws)	5. 120 feet (25 throws)
	6. Rest 10 minutes
	7. Warm-up throwing
	8. 120 feet (25 throws)

150-Foot Phase

Step 9	Step 10
1. Warm-up throwing	1. Warm-up throwing
2. 150 feet (25 throws)	2. 150 feet (25 throws)
3. Rest 15 minutes	3. Rest 10 minutes
4. Warm-up throwing	4. Warm-up throwing
5. 150 feet (25 throws)	5. 150 feet (25 throws)
	6. Rest 10 minutes
	7. Warm-up throwing
	8. 150 feet (25 throws)

position (Step 10). At that point, full strength should be restored in the athlete's arm. It is important to stress the crow-hop method and proper mechanics with each throw. Just as the advancement to this point has been gradual and progressive, the return to unrestricted throwing must follow the same principles. A pitcher should first throw only fast balls at 50%, progressing to 75% and then 100%. At that point, the player may start more stressful pitches, such as breaking balls. Other players should simulate a game situation, again progressing from 50% to 75% to 100%.

Once again, if an athlete has increased pain, particularly at the joint, the throwing program should be cut back and readvanced as tolerated, under the direction of the rehabilitation team.

In using the RSTP in conjunction with a structured rehabilitation program, the athlete should be able to return to full-competition status, minimizing any chance of reinjury. Program progression should be modified to meet the specific needs of the individual athlete. A comprehensive program consisting of a maintenance strength and flexibility program, appropriate warm-up and cooldown procedures, proper pitching mechanics, and progressive throwing and batting will assist the baseball player in returning safely to competition.

APPENDIX B

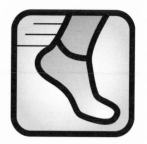

Return-to-Sport Tennis Program

- Begin at stage indicated by your therapist or doctor.

- Do not progress or continue program if joint pain is present.

- Always stretch your shoulder, elbow, and wrist before and after the interval program.

- Play on alternate days, giving your body a recovery day between sessions.

- Do not use a wall board, because it leads to exaggerated muscle contraction without rest between strokes.

- Ice your injured arm after each stage of the interval program.

- Have your stroke mechanics formally evaluated by a tennis teaching professional.

- Do not attempt to impart heavy topspin or underspin to your ground strokes until Stage 3 in the interval program.

- Contact your physical therapist or doctor if you have questions or problems with the interval program.

PERFORM EACH STAGE _____TIMES BEFORE PROGRESS-
ING TO THE NEXT STAGE. DO NOT PROGRESS TO THE
NEXT STAGE IF YOU HAD PAIN OR EXCESSIVE FATIGUE
ON YOUR PREVIOUS OUTING.

Step 1

a. Have a partner feed 20 forehand ground strokes to you from the
   net. (Partner must feed a slow, looping, waist-high feed.)

b. Have a partner feed 20 backhand ground strokes (as in Step 1a).

c. Rest 5 minutes.

d. Repeat 20 forehand and backhand feeds as above.

Step 2

a. Begin as in Step 1, with partner feeding 10 forehands and 10 backhands from the net.

b. Rally with partner from baseline, hitting controlled ground strokes
   until you have hit 25 strokes. (Alternate between forehand and
   backhand.)

c. Rest 5 minutes.

d. Repeat Step 2b.

Step 3

a. Rally ground strokes from baseline for 15 minutes.

b. Rest 5 minutes.

c. Hit 10 forehand and 10 backhand volleys, emphasizing a contact
   point in front of body.

d. Hit ground strokes from baseline for an additional 10 minutes.

e. Hit 10 forehand and 10 backhand volleys.

Step 4

a. Hit 20 minutes of ground strokes, mixing in volleys using a 70% ground strokes to 30% volleys format.

b. Hit 10 serves.

c. Rest 5 minutes.

d. Hit 10–15 more serves.

e. Finish with 5–10 minutes of ground strokes.

Step 5

a. Repeat Steps 4a and 4b, increasing the number of serves from 20 to 25 instead of 10–15.

b. Before resting, have a partner feed easy, short lobs to attempt a controlled overhead smash.

c. Repeat overhead 5–10 repetitions.

d. Finish with 5–10 minutes of ground strokes.

Step 6

a. Prior to attempting match play, complete Steps 1–5 without pain or excess fatigue in the upper extremity.

DO NOT PROGRESS FROM STAGE TO STAGE
IF PAIN DEVELOPS.

References

Achterberg, J. (1991, May). *Enhancing immune function through imagery.* Paper presented at the Fourth World Congress on Imagery, Minneapolis, MN.

Achterberg, J., Mathews-Simonton, S., & Simonton, O. C. (1977). Psychology of the exceptional cancer patient: A description of patients who outlive predicted life expectancies. *Psychotherapy: Theory, Research, and Practice, 14,* 416–422.

American Academy of Orthopaedic Surgeons. (1991). Physiology of tissue repair. In *Athletic training and sports medicine* (pp. 109–114). Park Ridge, IL: Author.

American Orthopaedic Society for Sports Medicine. (1999). *IKDC Subjective Knee Evaluation Form.* Retrieved October 21, 2002, from http://aclstudygroup.com/IKDC%20 form.htm#KDC%20SUBJECTIVE%20KNEE%20EVALUATION%20FORM

American Psychiatric Association. (1994). *Diagnostic and statistical manual of mental disorders* (4th ed.). Washington, DC: Author.

Andersen, M. B., & Williams, J. M. (1989, March). *Peripheral vision narrowing during stress: Possible mechanisms behind stress injury relationships.* Paper presented at the meeting of the Society of Behavioral Medicine, San Francisco.

Arnheim, D. D. (1986a). Emergency procedures. In D. A. Arnheim (Ed.), *Modern principles of athletic training* (pp. 263–264). St. Louis, MO: Times Mirror/Mosby.

Arnheim, D. D. (1986b). Tissue response to injury. In D. A. Arnheim (Ed.), *Modern principles of athletic training* (pp. 230–240). St. Louis, MO: Times Mirror/Mosby.

Arnheim, D. D. (1989). Exercise rehabilitation. In D. D. Arnheim (Ed.), *Modern principles of athletic training* (pp. 387–388). St. Louis, MO: Times/Mirror Mosby.

Ashton, C., Jr., Whitworth, G. C., Seldomridge, J. A., Shapiro, P. A., Weinberg, A. D., Michler, R. E., Smith, C. R., Rose, E. A., Fisher, S., & Oz, M. C. (1997). Self-hypnosis reduces anxiety following coronary artery bypass surgery. A prospective, randomized trial. *Journal of Cardiovascular Surgery, 38,* 69–75.

Ashton-Miller, J. A., Ottaviani, R. A., Hutchinson, C., & Wojtys, E. M. (1996). What best protects the inverted weightbearing ankle against further inversion? Evertor muscle strength compares favorably with shoe height, athletic tape, and three orthoses. *The American Journal of Sports Medicine, 6,* 800–809.

Asmundson, G. J. G., & Norton, G. R. (1995). Anxiety sensitivity in patients with physically unexplained chronic back pain: A preliminary report. *Behavior Research and Therapy, 33,* 771–777.

Atlee, J. L. (1999). *Complications in anesthesia*. Philadelphia: Saunders.

Avela, J., Kyrolainen, J., & Komi, P. (1999). Altered reflex sensitivity after repeated and prolonged passive muscle stretching. *Journal of Applied Physiology, 86*, 1283–1291.

Bandura, A. (1977). Self-efficacy: Toward a unifying theory of behavioral change. *Psychological Review, 84*, 191–215.

Barber, T. X. (1978). Hypnosis, suggestions, and psychosomatic phenomena: A new look from the standpoint of recent experimental studies. *The American Journal of Clinical Hypnosis, 21*, 13–27.

Beaton, D. E., & Richards, R. R. (1996). Measuring function of the shoulder. *Journal of Bone Joint Surgery, 78A*, 882–890.

Berntzen, D. (1987). Effects of multiple cognitive coping strategies on laboratory pain. *Cognitive Therapy and Research, 6*, 613–634.

Billig, N., Stockton, P., & Cohen-Mansfield, J. (1996). Cognitive and affective changes after cataract surgery in an elderly population. *American Journal of Geriatric Psychiatry, 4*, 29–38.

Bonci, C. M. (1999). Assessment and evaluation of predisposing factors to anterior cruciate ligament injury. *Journal of Athletic Training, 2*, 155–164.

Brewer, B. W. (1993). Self-identity and specific vulnerability to depressed mood. *Journal of Personality, 61*, 343–364.

Brewer, B. W. (1994). Review and critique of models of psychological adjustment to athletic injury. *Journal of Applied Sport Psychology, 6*, 87–100.

Brewer, B. W., Cornelius, A. E., Van Raalte, J. L., Petitpas, A. J., Sklar, J. H., Pohlman, M. H., Krushell, R. J., & Ditmar, T. D. (1998, August). *Previous surgical experience and anxiety prior to anterior cruciate ligament reconstruction: Ignorance is bliss?* Paper presented at the 24th International Congress of Applied Psychology, San Francisco.

Brewer, B. W., Jeffers, K. E., Petitpas, A. J., & Van Raalte, J. L. (1994). Perceptions of psychological interventions in the context of sport injury rehabilitation. *The Sport Psychologist, 8*, 176–188.

Brewer, B. W., Linder, D. E., & Phelps, C. M. (1995). Situational correlates of emotional adjustment to athletic injury. *Clinical Journal of Sports Medicine, 5*, 241–245.

Brewer, B. W., Petitpas, A. J., Van Raalte, J. L., Sklar, J. H., & Ditmar, T. D. (1995). Prevalence of psychological distress among patients at a physical therapy clinic specializing in sports medicine. *Sports Medicine, Training, and Rehabilitation, 6*, 139–145.

Brewer, B. W., & Petrie, T. A. (1995, Spring). A comparison between injured and uninjured football players on selected psychosocial variables. *The Academic Athletic Journal*, pp. 11–17.

Brewer, B. W., Van Raalte, J. L., & Linder, D. E. (1991). Role of the sport psychologist in treating injured athletes: A survey of sports medicine providers. *Journal of Applied Sport Psychology, 3*, 183–190.

Brewer, B. W., Van Raalte, J. L., & Linder, D. E. (1993). Athletic identity: Hercules' muscles or Achilles heel? *International Journal of Sport Psychology, 24*, 237–254.

Brownstein, B., & Bronner, S. (1997). *Functional movement in orthopaedic and sports physical therapy*. Philadelphia: Churchill Livingstone.

Bunker, L., Williams, J. M., & Zinsser, N. (1993). Cognitive techniques for improving performance and building confidence. In J. M. Williams (Ed.), *Applied sport psychology: Personal growth to peak performance* (2nd ed., pp. 225–242). Palo Alto, CA: Mayfield.

Byerly, P. N., Worrell, T., Gahimer, J., & Domholdt, E. (1994). Rehabilitation compliance in an athletic training environment. *Journal of Athletic Training, 29*, 352–355.

Cautela, J. R., & Wisocki, P. A. (1977). Thought-stopping procedure: Description, application, and learning theory interpretations. *Psychological Records, 27*, 255–264.

Cawley, P. W. (2000). Bracing: Science or psychology? In T. S. Ellenbecker (Ed.), *Knee ligament rehabilitation* (pp. 252–261). Philadelphia: Churchill Livingstone.

Chaudhury, S., Chakraborty, P. K., Gurunadh, V. S., & Ratha, P. (1997). Emotional reactions to cataract surgery with intraocular lens implantation. *Journal of Personality and Clinical Studies, 13*, 39–43.

Clark, I. V. (1960). Effects of mental practice on the development of a certain motor skill. *The Research Quarterly, 31*, 560–569.

Clayman, C. B. (1989). *The American Medical Association home medical encyclopedia.* New York: Random House.

Cohen, L. H. (1988). *Life events and psychological functioning: Theoretical and methodological issues.* Newbury Park, CA: Sage.

Cousins, M. J., & Phillips, G. D. (Eds.). (1985). *Acute pain management. Clinics in critical care medicine series: Vol. 8.* New York: Churchill.

Crossman, J., & Jamieson, J. (1985). Differences in perceptions of seriousness and disrupting effects of athletic injury as viewed by athletes and their trainer. *Perceptual and Motor Skills, 61*, 1131–1134.

Daly, J. M., Brewer, B. W., Van Raalte, J. L., Petitpas, A. J., & Sklar, J. H. (1995). Cognitive appraisal, emotional adjustment, and adherence to rehabilitation following knee surgery. *Journal of Sport Rehabilitation, 4*, 23–30.

Davies, G. J. (1992). *A compendium of isokinetics in clinical usage* (4th ed.). Lacrosse, WI: S & S.

Davies, G. J., & Zillmer, D. A. (2000). Functional progression of exercise in rehabilitation. In T. S. Ellenbecker (Ed.), *Knee ligament rehabilitation* (pp. 345–357). Philadelphia: Churchill Livingstone.

Derscheid, G. L., & Feiring, D. C. (1987). A statistical analysis to characteristic treatment adherence of the 18 most common diagnoses seen at a sports medicine clinic. *Journal of Orthopaedics and Sports Physical Therapy, 9*, 40–46.

Duda, J. L., Smart, A. E., & Tappe, M. K. (1989). Predictors of adherence in the rehabilitation of athletic injuries: An application of personal investment theory. *Journal of Sport and Exercise Psychology, 11*, 367–381.

Duits, A. A., Duivenvoorden, H. J., Boeke, S., Taams, M. A., Mochtar, B., Krauss, X. H., Passchier, J., & Erdman, R. A. (1999). A structural modeling analysis of anxiety and depression in patients undergoing coronary artery bypass graft surgery: A model generating approach. *Journal of Psychosomatic Research, 46*, 187–200.

The essential guide to vitamins and minerals. (1995). New York: HarperCollins.

Eysenck, H. J. (1994). Cancer, personality, and stress: Prediction and prevention. *Advances in Behaviour Research and Therapy, 16,* 167–215.

Feltz, D. L. (1986). The psychology of sports injuries. In P. E. Vinger & E. F. Hoerner (Eds.), *Sports injuries: The unthwarted epidemic* (2nd ed., pp. 336–344). Boston: John Wright, PSG.

Fernandez, E., & Turk, D. C. (1986, August). *Overall and relative efficacy of cognitive strategies in attenuating pain.* Paper presented at the 94th annual convention of the American Psychological Association, Washington, DC.

Ferrell-Torry, A. T., & Glick, O. J. (1993). The use of therapeutic massage as a nursing intervention to modify anxiety and the perception of cancer pain. *Cancer Nursing, 16,* 93–101.

Fiore, N. A. (1988). The inner healer: Imagery for coping with cancer and its therapy. *Journal of Mental Imagery, 12,* 79–82.

Fisher, A. C., Mullins, S. A., & Frye, P. A. (1993). Athletic trainers' attitudes and judgments of injured athletes' rehabilitation adherence. *Journal of Athletic Training, 28,* 43–47.

Fleck, S., & Kraemer, W. (1986). *Designing resistance training programs.* Champaign, IL: Human Kinetics.

Fleisig, G. S., Andrews, J. R., Dillman, C. J., & Escamilla, R. F. (1995). Kinetics of baseball pitching with implications about injury mechanisms. *American Journal of Sports Medicine, 23,* 233–239.

Fortner, P. A. (1998). Preoperative patient preparation: Psychological and educational aspects. *Seminars in Perioperative Nursing, 7,* 3–9.

Franco, K., Tamburino, M., Campbell, N., Zrull, J., Evans, C., & Bronson, D. (1995). The added costs of depression to medical care. *Pharmacoeconomics, 7,* 284–291.

Fredrikson, M., Furst, C. J., Ekander, M., & Rotstein, S. (1993). Trait anxiety and anticipatory immune reactions in women receiving adjuvant chemotherapy for breast cancer. *Brain, Behavior, & Immunity, 7,* 79–90.

Furlong, M. W. (2000). Anesthesia. *Microsoft® Encarta® online encyclopedia* [On-line]. Available: http://www.encarta.msn.com

Ganster, D. C., & Victor, B. (1988). The impact of social support on mental and physical health. *British Journal of Medical Psychology, 61,* 17–36.

Gaston, L., Crombez, J., & Dupuis, G. (1989). An imagery and meditation technique in the treatment of psoriasis: A case study using an A-B-A design. *Journal of Mental Imagery, 13,* 31–38.

Giesecke, M. E. (1987). The symptom of insomnia in university students. *Journal of American College Health, 35,* 215–221.

Gipson, M., Foster, M., Yaffe, D., O'Carroll, V., Bene, C., & Moore, B. (1989, April). *Opportunities for health psychology in medicine services and training.* Paper presented at the Western Psychological Association/Rocky Mountain Psychological Association Joint Annual Convention, Reno, NV.

Goats, G. C. (1994). Massage—The scientific basis for an ancient art: Parts 1 and 2. *British Journal of Sports Medicine, 28,* 149–152, 153–156.

Gordon, S., Milios, D., & Grove, J. R. (1991). Psychological aspects of the recovery process from sport injury: The perspective of sport physiotherapists. *Australian Journal of Science and Medicine in Sport, 23,* 53–60.

Gould, D. (1993). Goal setting for peak performance. In J. Williams (Ed.), *Applied sport psychology: Personal growth to peak performance* (pp. 158–169). Palo Alto, CA: Mayfield.

Granito, V. J., Hogan, J. B., & Varnum, L. K. (1995). The Performance Enhancement Group program: Integrating sport psychology and rehabilitation. *Journal of Athletic Training, 30,* 328–331.

Green, L. B. (1992). The use of imagery in the rehabilitation of injured athletes. *The Sport Psychologist, 6,* 416–428.

Greenspan, M. J., & Feltz, D. L. (1989). Psychological interventions with athletes in competitive situations: A review. *The Sport Psychologist, 3,* 219–236.

Gregory, W., Cialdini, R., & Carpenter, K. (1982). Self-reliant scenarios as mediators of likelihood estimates and compliance: Does imagining make it so? *Journal of Personality and Social Psychology, 43,* 89–99.

Grove, J. R., & Gordon, A. M. D. (1992). The psychological aspects of injury in sport. In J. Bloomfield, P. A. Fricker, & K. D. Fitch (Eds.), *Textbook of science and medicine in sport* (pp. 176–186). Carlton, Victoria, Australia: Blackwell Scientific.

Guide to physical therapy practice. (1997). *Physical Therapy, 77,* 1163–1650.

Hackfort, D., & Schwenkmezger, P. (1993). Anxiety. In R. N. Singer, M. Murphey, & L. K. Tennant (Eds.), *Handbook on research on sport psychology* (pp. 328–364). New York: Macmillan.

Harrelson, G. L., Weber, M. D., & Leaver-Dunn, D. (1998). Use of modalities in rehabiliation. In J. R. Andrews, K. E. Wilk, & G. L. Harrelson (Eds.), *Physical rehabilitation of the injured athlete* (2nd ed., pp. 82–145). Philadelphia: Saunders.

Harris, D. V., & Williams, J. M. (1993). Relaxation and energizing techniques for regulation of arousal. In J. Williams (Ed.), *Applied sport psychology* (pp. 185–199). Mountain View, CA: Mayfield.

Heil, J. (1993). *Psychology of sport injury.* Champaign, IL: Human Kinetics.

Hellstedt, J. C. (1987). Sport psychology at a ski academy: Teaching mental skills to young athletes. *The Sport Psychologist, 1,* 56–68.

Hewett, T. E. (1998). Cincinnati Sportsmetrics: A training program for the preventions of knee injuries in female athletes. *Sports and Medicine Today, 1,* 63–66.

Ho, S. S., Coel, M. N., Kagawa, R., & Richardson, A. B. (1994). The effects of ice on blood flow and bone metabolism in knees. *American Journal of Sports Medicine, 4,* 537–540.

Ho, S. S., Coel, M. N., Kagawa, R., & Richardson, A. B. (1995). Comparison of various icing times in decreasing bone metabolism and blood flow in the knee. *American Journal of Sports Medicine, 23,* 74–76.

Holden-Lund, C. (1988). Effects of relaxation with guided imagery on surgical stress and wound healing. *Research in Nursing and Health, 11,* 235–244.

Huo, M. H., & Harrison, R. J. (2000, April). Management game plan helps thwart thromboembolism. *Biomechanics,* pp. 37–42.

Ievleva, L., & Orlick, T. (1991). Mental links to enhancing healing: An exploratory study. *The Sport Psychologist, 5,* 25–40.

Ireland, M. L. (1999). Anterior cruciate ligament injury in female athletes: Epidemiology. *Journal of Athletic Training, 2,* 150–154.

Israel, S. (1976). Zur problematik des uebertrainings aus internistischer und leistungs-physioligischer sicht [The problem of overtraining from the perspective of internal medicine and exercise physiology]. *Medizin und Sport, 16,* 1–12.

Jacobson, E. (1938). *Progressive relaxation: A physiological and clinical investigation of muscular states and their significance in psychology and medical practice.* Chicago: University of Chicago Press.

Kaard, B., & Tostinbo, O. (1989). Increase on plasma beta endorphins in a connective tissue massage. *General Pharmacology, 20,* 487–489.

Kiecolt-Glaser, J. K., Page, G. G., Marucha, P. T., MacCallum, R. C., & Glaser, R. (1998). Stress and immune functioning. *American Psychologist, 53,* 1209–1218.

Kindermann, W. (1988). Metabolic and hormonal reactions in overtraining. *Seminars in Orthopaedics, 3,* 207–216.

King, P. (1996, July 15). Five questions. *Sports Illustrated, 85,* 74–79.

Kirkendall, D. T., & Garrett, W. E., Jr., (2000). The anterior cruciate enigma. *Clinical Orthopaedics and Related Research, 372,* 64–68.

Kokkonen, J., Nelson, A. G., & Cornwell, A. (1998). Acute muscle stretching inhibits maximal strength performance. *Research Quarterly of Exercise and Sport, 69,* 411–415.

Korn, E. R. (1983). The use of altered states of consciousness and imagery in physical and pain rehabilitation. *Journal of Mental Imagery, 7,* 25–34.

Kuipers, H., & Keizer, H. A. (1988). Overtraining in elite athletes: Review and directions for the future. *Sports Medicine, 6,* 79–92.

Kulik, J. A., & Mahler, H. I. (1993). Emotional support as a moderator of adjustment and compliance after coronary artery bypass surgery: A longitudinal study. *Journal of Behavioral Medicine, 16,* 45–63.

Kurlowicz, L. H. (1998). Perceived self-efficacy, functional ability, and depressive symptoms in older elective surgery patients. *Nursing Research, 47,* 219–226.

Lang, P. J. (1977). Imagery in therapy: An information-processing analysis of fear. *Behavior Therapy, 8,* 862–886.

Langer, E. J., Janis, I. L., & Wolfer, J. A. (1975). Reduction of psychological stress in surgical patients. *Journal of Experimental Social Psychology, 11,* 155–165.

Larson, G. A., Starkey, C., & Zaichkowsky, L. D. (1996). Psychological aspects of athletic injuries as perceived by athletic trainers. *The Sport Psychologist, 10,* 37–47.

Leddy, M., Lambert, M., & Ogles, B. (1994). Psychological consequences of athletic injury among high-level competitors. *Research Quarterly, 65,* 347–354.

Lee, J. (1993). Psychological disturbances and an exaggerated response to pain in patients with whiplash injury. *Journal of Psychosomatic Research, 37,* 105–110.

Lephart, S. M., Henry, T. J., Riemann, B. L., Giannantonio, F. P., & Fu, F. H. (1998). The effects of neuromuscular control exercises on functional stability in the unstable shoulder. *Journal of Athletic Training, 33,* 515.

Lindenfeld, T. N. (1998, April). Recognizing and managing reflex sympathetic dystrophy. *The Journal of Musculoskeletal Medicine, 15*, 41–53.

Lindenfeld, T. N., Wojtys, E. M., & Husain, A. (1999). Operative treatment of arthrofibrosis of the knee. *The Journal of Bone and Joint Surgery, 81-A*, 1772–1783.

Linder, D. E., Pillow, D. R., & Reno, R. R. (1989). Shrinking jocks: Derogation of athletes who consult a sport psychologist. *Journal of Sport and Exercise Psychology, 11*, 270–280.

Locke, E. A., Shaw, K. N., Saari, L. M., & Latham, G. P. (1981). Goal setting and task performance. *Psychological Bulletin, 90*, 125–152.

Logsdon, M. C., Usui, W. M., Cronin, S. N., & Miracle, V. A. (1998). Social support and adjustment in women following coronary artery bypass surgery. *Health Care for Women International, 19*, 61–70.

Marshall, R. N., Noffal, G. L., & Legnanni, G. (1993). Simulation of the tennis serve: Factors affecting elbow torques related to medial epicondylitis. In *Biomechanics* (pp. 88–99). Paris: ISB.

McConnell, J. (2000). Patellofemoral joint complications and considerations. In T. S. Ellenbecker (Ed.), *Knee ligament rehabilitation* (pp. 202–224). Philadelphia: Churchill Livingstone.

McDonald, S. A., & Hardy, C. J. (1990). Affective response patterns of the injured athlete: An exploratory analysis. *The Sport Psychologist, 4*, 261–274.

McGee, P. (1998). Training may reduce knee injuries for female athletes. *Orthopedics Today, 9*, 12–16.

Meichenbaum, D. (1985). *Stress inoculation training.* New York: Pergamon Press.

Meichenbaum, D., & Turk, D. C. (1987). *Facilitating treatment adherence: A practitioner's guidebook.* New York: Plenum.

Miles, M. S. (1985). Emotional symptoms and physical health in bereaved parents. *Nursing Research, 34*, 76–81.

Morgan, W. P., & Pollock, M. L. (1977). Psychological characterization of the elite distance runner. *Annals of the New York Academy of Science, 301*, 382–403.

Navateur, J. (1992). Anxiety, emotion, and cerebral blood flow. *International Journal of Psychophysiology, 13*, 137–146.

Nelson, F. V., Zimmerman, L., Barnason, S., Nieveen, J., & Schmaderer, M. (1998). The relationship and influence of anxiety on postoperative pain in the coronary artery bypass patient. *Journal of Pain and Symptom Management, 15*, 102–109.

Nideffer, R. M. (1976). Test of attentional and interpersonal style. *Journal of Personality and Social Psychology, 34*, 394–404.

Nideffer, R. M. (1983). The injury athlete: Psychological factors in treatment. *Orthopedic Clinics of North America, 14*, 372–385.

Nideffer, R. M. (1989). Theoretical and practical relationships between attention, anxiety, and performance in sports. In D. Hackfort & C. D. Spielberger (Eds.), *Anxiety in sport: An international perspective* (pp. 117–136). New York: Hemisphere.

Orbell, S., Johnston, M., Rowley, D., Espley, A., & Davey, P. (1998). Cognitive representations of illness and functional and affective adjustment following surgery for osteoarthritis. *Social Science and Medicine, 47*, 93–102.

Palimitier, R. A., An, K. K., Scott, S. G., & Chao, E. Y. S. (1991). Kinetic chain exercises in knee rehabilitation. *Sports Medicine, 11*, 402–413.

Parent, N. (1997). Social support interventions by former model patients for persons undergoing heart surgery. *Recherche en Soins Infirmiers, 51*, 59–100.

Pearson, L., & Jones, G. (1992). Emotional effects of sports injuries: Implications for physiotherapists. *Physiotherapy, 78*, 762–770.

Perski, A., Feleke, E., Anderson, G., Samad, B. A., Westerlund, H., Ericsson, C. G., & Rehnqvist, N. (1998). Emotional distress before coronary bypass grafting limits the benefits of surgery. *American Heart Journal, 136*, 510–517.

Pines, A. M., Aronson, E., & Kafry, D. (1981). *Burnout.* New York: Free Press.

Pollard, H. (1994). Athletic injuries: A psychological perspective to rehabilitation. *Chiropractic Sports Medicine, 8*, 18–31.

Post-White, J. (1991, May). *The effects of mental imagery on emotions, immune function, and cancer outcome.* Paper presented at the Fourth World Congress on Imagery, Minneapolis, MN.

Prentice, W. E. (1986). Intermittent compression devices. In W. E. Prentice (Ed.), *Therapeutic modalities in sports medicine* (pp. 207–212). St. Louis, MO: Times Mirror/Mosby.

Prentice, W. E. (1999). Using therapeutic modalities in rehabilitation. In W. E. Prentice (Ed.), *Rehabilitation techniques in sports medicine* (pp. 238–240). Boston: McGraw-Hill.

Richman, J. M., Hardy, C. J., Rosenfeld, L. B., & Callanan, R. A. E. (1989). Strategies for enhancing social support networks in sport: A brainstorming experience. *Journal of Applied Sport Psychology, 1*, 150–159.

Rochman, S. (1996). Gender inequality. *Training and Conditioning, 6*, 10–20.

Roetert, E. P., & Ellenbecker, T. S. (1998). *Complete conditioning for tennis.* Champaign, IL: Human Kinetics.

Rosenfeld, L. B., Richman, J. M., & Hardy, C. J. (1989). An examination of social support networks among athletes: Description and relationship to stress. *The Sport Psychologist, 3*, 23–33.

Rotella, R. J., & Heyman, S. R. (1993). Stress, injury, and the psychological rehabilitation of athletes. In J. Williams (Ed.), *Applied sport psychology* (pp. 338–355). Mountain View, CA: Mayfield.

Sarason, I. G., Sarason, B. R., & Pierce, G. R. (1990). Social support, personality, and performance. *Journal of Applied Sport Psychology, 2*, 117–127.

Sarno, J. (1984). *Mind over back pain.* New York: Morrow.

Schonfeld, L. (1992). Covert assertion as a method of coping with pain and pain related behaviors. *Clinical Gerontologist, 12*, 17–29.

Schurman, D. J., Goodman, S. B., & Smith, R. L. (1990). Inflammation and tissue repair. In W. B. Leadbetter, J. A. Buckwalter, & S. L. Gordon (Eds.), *Sports induced inflammation* (pp. 277–282). Park Ridge, IL: American Academy of Orthopaedic Surgeons.

Sheikh, A. A., & Jordan, C. S. (1983). Clinical uses of mental imagery. In A. A. Sheikh (Ed.), *Imagery: Current theory, research, and applications* (pp. 391–435). New York: Wiley.

Shelbourne, K. D., & Wilckens, J. H. (1990). Current concepts in anterior cruciate ligament rehabilitation. *Orthopaedic Review, 19*, 957–964.

Shellock, F., Mullin, M. J., Stone, K. R., & Coleman, M. (2000). Development and clinical application of kinematic MRI of the patellofemoral joint using an extremity MR system. *Journal of Athletic Training, 3,* 12–16.

Smith, D. (1987). Conditions that facilitate the development of sport imagery training. *The Sport Psychologist, 1,* 237–247.

Smith, R. L., & Brunolli, J. (1989). Shoulder kinesthesia after anterior glenohumeral joint dislocation. *Physical Therapy, 69,* 106–112.

Somer, E. (1995). Vitamins and minerals in the body. In *The essential guide to vitamins and minerals.* New York: HarperCollins.

Steadman, J. R. (1982). Rehabilitation of skiing injuries. *Clinics in Sports Medicine, 1,* 289–294.

Steadman, J. R. (1993). A physician's approach to the psychology of injury. In J. Heil (Ed.), *Psychology of sport injury* (pp. 25–31). Champaign, IL: Human Kinetics.

Street still haunted by accident. (1998, September 22). *The Denver Post,* p. 12D.

Suinn, R. (1993). Imagery. In R. N. Singer, M. Murphey, & L. K. Tennant (Eds.), *Handbook on research on sport psychology* (pp. 492–510). New York: Macmillan.

Szeverenyi, P., Bacsko, G., Hetey, M., Kovacsne, T. Z., Csiszar, P., Korosi, T., & Borsos, A. (1999). The healing process following gynecologic laparoscopy: Date on the significance of psychological factors. *Orvosi Hetilap, 140,* 1043–1048.

Taylor, J. (2001). *Prime sport: Triumph of the athlete mind.* New York: Universe.

Taylor, J., Horevitz, R., & Balague, G. (1993). The use of hypnosis in applied sport psychology. *The Sport Psychologist, 7,* 58–78.

Taylor, S. E., Falke, R. L., Shoptaw, S. J., & Lichtman, R. R. (1986). Social support groups and the cancer patient. *Journal of Consulting and Clinical Psychology, 54,* 608–615.

Taylor, J., & Taylor, S. (1997). *Psychological approaches to sports injury rehabilitation.* Austin, TX: PRO-ED.

Tegner, Y., & Lysolm, J. (1985). Rating systems in the evaluation of knee ligament injuries. *Clinical Orthopaedics and Related Research, 198,* 43–49.

Teitz, C. C., Hu, S. S., & Arendt, E. A. (1997). The female athlete: Evaluation and treatment of sports-related problems. *Journal of the American Academy of Orthopaedic Surgeons, 2,* 91–92.

Tharp, G. D., & Barnes, M. W. (1989). Reduction of immunoglobulin-A by swim training. *Medicine and Science in Sports and Exercise, 21*(Suppl.), 109.

Timberlake, N., Klinger, L., Smith, P., Venn, G., Treasure, T., Harrison, M., & Newman, S. P. (1997). Incidence and patterns of depression following coronary artery bypass graft surgery. *Journal of Psychosomatic Research, 43,* 197–207.

Tricker, R., & Cook, D. L. (1990). *Athletes at risk: Drugs and sports.* Dubuque, IA: Wm. C. Brown.

Tversky, A., & Kahneman, D. (1973). Availability: A heuristic for judging frequency and probability. *Cognitive Psychology, 5,* 207–232.

Vealey, R. S., & Walter, S. M. (1993). Imagery training for performance enhancement and personal development. In J. Williams (Ed.), *Applied sport psychology* (pp. 200–224). Mountain View, CA: Mayfield.

Vingerhoets, G. (1998a). Cognitive, emotional, and psychosomatic complaints and their relation to emotional status and personality following cardiac surgery. *British Journal of Health Psychology, 3,* 159–169.

Vingerhoets, G. (1998b). Perioperative anxiety and depression in open-heart surgery. *Psychosomatics, 39,* 30–37.

Wack, J. T., & Turk, D. C. (1984). Latent structures in strategies for coping with pain. *Health Psychology, 3,* 27–43.

Weiner, R. (1998, July 21). Rice is "running scared." *USA Today,* pp. 1–2C.

Weiss, M. R., & Troxel, R. K. (1986). Psychology of the injured athlete. *Athletic Training, 21,* 104–154.

Weltman, G., & Egstrom, G. H. (1966). Perceptual narrowing in novice divers. *Human Factors, 8,* 499–506.

Wiese, D. M., & Weiss, M. R. (1987). Psychology rehabilitation and physical injury: Implications for the sports medicine team. *The Sport Psychologist, 1,* 318–330.

Wiese, D. M., Weiss, M. R., & Yukelson, D. P. (1991). Sport psychology in the training room: A survey of athletic trainers. *The Sport Psychologist, 5,* 15–24.

Wilk, K. E. (1999). Rehabilitation after anterior cruciate ligament reconstruction in the female athlete. *Journal of Athletic Training, 2,* 181–182.

Wilk, K. E., & Andrews, J. R. (1997). *Interval throwing program.* Birmingham, AL: American Sports Medicine Institute.

Williams, J. M., & Roepke, N. (1993). Psychology of injury and injury rehabilitation. In R. N. Singer, M. Murphey, & L. K. Tennant (Eds.), *Handbook of research on sport psychology* (pp. 815–839). New York: Macmillan.

Wojtys, E. M., Kothari, S. U., & Huston, L. J. (1996). Anterior cruciate ligament functional brace use in sports. *The American Journal of Sports Medicine, 4,* 539–546.

Woolfolk, R., Parrish, W., & Murphy, S. M. (1985). The effects of positive and negative imagery on motor skill performance. *Cognitive Therapy and Research, 9,* 235–241.

Youmans, S. (1999, August 27). Study: Women troubled more by knee injuries. *Hartford Courant,* p. B7.

Zachezewski, J. E., & Reischl, S. (1986). Flexibility for the runner: Specific program considerations. *Topics in Acute Care and Trauma Rehabilitation, 1,* 9–27.

Zanolla, R., Monzeglio, C., & Balzarini, A. (1984). Evaluation of the results of three different methods of postmastectomy lymphedema treatment. *Journal of Surgical Oncology, 26,* 210–213.

Index

About the Authors

Jim Taylor, PhD, is internationally recognized for his work in the psychology of sport and injury rehabilitation. He has been a consultant to the United States and Japanese Ski Teams, USA Triathlon, and the United States Tennis Association, and has worked with healthy and injured athletes in the NFL, NBA, MLB, PGA, ATP, and WTA, and with athletes at all levels of ability in many sports. Dr. Taylor has consulted with the Mayo Clinic, the Stone Clinic in San Francisco, the Aspen Valley Hospital, and the Aspen Fitness and Sports Medicine Institute.

Dr. Taylor is a former associate professor in the School of Psychology at Nova University in Fort Lauderdale and is currently President of Alpine/Taylor Consulting, a performance psychology consulting firm in San Francisco. A former U.S. top-20 ranked alpine ski racer who competed internationally, Dr. Taylor is also a United States Professional Tennis Association certified tennis-teaching professional, a second-degree black belt and certified instructor in karate, a marathon runner, and Ironman triathlete.

Dr. Taylor is the author of 7 books including the *Prime Sport* book series, *Psychological Approaches to Sports Injury Rehabilitation*, and *Psychology of Dance*. He has published over 300 articles in professional and popular publications and serves on the editorial boards of several scholarly journals. Dr. Taylor has given more than 400 workshops and presentations throughout North America and Europe.

Kevin R. Stone, MD, is an orthopedic surgeon and chairman of The Stone Foundation for Sports Medicine and Arthritis Research at The Stone Clinic in San Francisco. He specializes in sports medicine with a special interest in knee and shoulder injuries. He has lectured internationally as an expert in cartilage and meniscal growth, replacement, and repair.

250

Dr. Stone is a physician for the U.S. Ski Team, the Lawrence Pech Dance Company, the Marin Ballet, and the Smuin Ballet. He has served as a physician for the U.S. Pro Ski Tour, the Old Blues Rugby Club, the modern pentathlon at the U.S. Olympic Festival, and the United States Olympic Training Center.

Dr. Stone founded The Stone Foundation for Sports Medicine and Arthritis Research in 1995 to evaluate research at The Stone Clinic in San Francisco. The foundation conducts research in advanced surgical techniques for orthopedic sports medicine. These efforts have led to improvements in cartilage replacement and regeneration, cruciate ligament repair and reconstruction, and techniques to prevent osteoarthritic degeneration.

Michael J. Mullin, ATC, PTA, is the head clinical athletic trainer at Healthsouth/Orthopaedic Associates in Portland, Maine, an orthopedic surgery and rehabilitation facility. With over 10 years of experience in sports medicine, Mr. Mullin has worked with numerous sports and activities providing athletic therapy, physical training, and conditioning services. He has served as head athletic therapist for the Lawrence Pech Dance Company, the Smuin Ballet, and the Marin Ballet. Mr. Mullin has provided athletic training services for the national champion Old Blues Rugby Club and the U.S. Windsurfing Association National Championships, and has overseen physical conditioning camps and rehabilitation services for athletes of the U.S. Ski Team and the World Pro Ski Tour.

He is a sports medicine and fitness consultant for numerous magazines including *Shape, Women's Sports and Fitness, Men's Fitness, Skiing*, and *Windsurfing*. Mr. Mullin is a clinic advisor for the American Running and Fitness Association and also serves on the editorial board for the *Sports Medicine and Athletic Training Patient Education Manual*. He lectures regularly and frequently publishes articles about training and conditioning principles, injury prevention, and rehabilitation.

Todd Ellenbecker, MS, PT, SCS, OCS, CSCS, is a physical therapist and clinic director of Physiotherapy Associates Scottsdale Sports Clinic in Scottsdale, Arizona. He is a certified sports clinical specialist and orthopedic clinical specialist by the American Physical Therapy Association (APTA), and a certified strength and conditioning specialist. Mr. Ellenbecker is a United States Professional Tennis Association certified tennis teaching professional and a member of the United States Tennis Association Sport Science Committee.

Mr. Ellenbecker is the chairman of the APTA's Shoulder Special Interest Group and a manuscript reviewer for the *Journal of Orthopaedic and Sports Physical Therapy*. He is also on the editorial board of the *Journal of Strength and Conditioning Research*. Mr. Ellenbecker has conducted and published research primarily on upper extremity athletes as well as on open- and closed-chain rehabilitation for the upper and lower extremities. He has conducted research and lectured internationally on shoulder and elbow rehabilitation as well as isokinetic exercise application and reliability. Mr. Ellenbecker is the author of two books, *The Elbow in Sport* and *Complete Conditioning for Tennis*, and is the editor of *Knee Ligament Rehabilitation*.

Ann Walgenbach, RNC, FNP, MSN, ONC, CNOR, RNFA, is a family nurse practitioner at The Stone Clinic in San Francisco. She is the initial interviewer of patients at the clinic, the first surgical assistant to Dr. Kevin Stone in surgery, and involved in the research conducted by The Stone Foundation for Sports Medicine and Arthritis Research. Ms. Walgenbach is a certified orthopedic nurse, certified operating room nurse, and certified RN First Assistant.

Ms. Walgenbach has been a registered nurse for 21 years. She worked at UCLA Medical Center for 10 years on the surgical floor and then in the trauma/neurosurgery intensive care unit. Ms. Walgenbach earned her MS in nursing from UCLA and, in 1992, joined The Stone Clinic staff to focus on a more wellness-oriented form of health care.

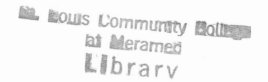